AIR FRYER

Cookbook for a Healthy Life

(Delicious Recipes for Hassle-free Cooking)

Johnny Shaw

Published by Alex Howard

© Johnny Shaw

All Rights Reserved

Air Fryer: Cookbook for a Healthy Life (Delicious Recipes for Hassle-free Cooking)

ISBN 978-1-989891-80-3

All rights reserved. No part of this guide may be reproduced in any form without permission in writing from the publisher except in the case of brief quotations embodied in critical articles or reviews.

Legal & Disclaimer

The information contained in this book is not designed to replace or take the place of any form of medicine or professional medical advice. The information in this book has been provided for educational and entertainment purposes only.

The information contained in this book has been compiled from sources deemed reliable, and it is accurate to the best of the Author's knowledge; however, the Author cannot guarantee its accuracy and validity and cannot be held liable for any errors or omissions. Changes are periodically made to this book. You must consult your doctor or get professional medical advice before using any of the suggested remedies, techniques, or information in this book.

Table of Contents

PART 1 .... **9**

CHAPTER 1: INTRODUCTION **10**

CHAPTER 2: BREAKFAST SWEETS **11**

    CINNAMON AND SUGAR DONUTS 11
    BLUEBERRY MUFFINS 13
    DOUBLE THE CHOCOLATE MUFFINS 14
    CINNAMON OR VANILLA FRENCH TOAST STICKS 15
    PLAIN DONUTS WITH STRAWBERRY ICING 16
    CHOCOLATE ECLAIRS 17
    BREAKFAST OR TEA TIME SCONES 19

CHAPTER 3: COOKIES AND BROWNIES **20**

    CHOCOLATE BROWNIES 20
    OATMEAL RAISIN COOKIES 21
    CHOCOLATE CHIP COOKIES 22
    PEANUT BUTTER COOKIES 23
    SNICKERDOODLES 24
    CHEESECAKE SWIRL BROWNIES 25
    MINT CHOCOLATE BROWNIES 26

CHAPTER 4: CAKES AND CUPCAKES **28**

    RED VELVET CUPCAKES 28
    DREAMY CHOCOLATE CAKE 29
    MARVELOUS MARBLE CAKE 30
    AMAZING MOLTEN LAVA CAKE 31
    CARROT CAKE WITH CREAM CHEESE FROSTING 33
    HAPPY BIRTHDAY CAKE 35
    VANILLA CHIFFON CAKE 36

CHAPTER 5: FRUIT-FILLED GOODNESS **37**

    BANANA BREAD 37
    MINI PUMPKIN PIES 38
    SCRUMPTIOUS APPLE PIE 40
    FANTASMIC FRUIT JAM TARTS 41
    CINNAMON APPLE SAMOSAS 42
    LOVELY LEMON BARS 43
    RAISIN BREAD PUDDING 44

CONCLUSION **45**

PART 2 .... **46**

INTRODUCTION **47**

WHAT ARE THE BENEFITS OF AN AIR FRYER? **47**

IS IT AS HEALTHY AS YOU THINK? **49**

FRYER WITHOUT OIL WHICH ONE TO BUY? 50
    WHAT SHOULD YOU KEEP IN MIND BEFORE BUYING AN AIR FRYER 53

AIR FRYER VS. OVEN 54

AIR FRYER RECIPES 56

1. Fish in Air Fryer 56
2. Wings in air fryer 57
3. Gluten-free yogurt cake in air fryer 57
4. Mini Tatin cake in the air fryer 58
5. Rabas in hot air fryer 58
6. Spanish potatoes in hot air fryer 59
7. Breaded prawns in hot air fryer 59
8. Pizzetas in fryer without oil 60
9. Wings with fine herbs without oil (in the fryer without oil) 61
10. Bondiola chopped (air fryer) 61
11. Zucchini sticks in oil-free fryer / oven 62
12. Pumpkin croquettes using oil-free fryer 62
13. 4D turbocecofry iron knives, dietary fryer 63
14. Spiced chicken wings, in oil-free fryer 63
15. Grilled squid with jocca oil-free fryer 64
16. French fries and Iberian pork fillets in a fryer without jocca oil 64
17. Roasted apples in Jocca oil-free fryer 65
18. Chard fritters with Electric Fryer 65
19. Chicken fajitas 66
20. Fried cheese 67
21. Chicken fingers 67
22. Cod fillet, and cocorita purslane sauce 68
23. Stew Italian zucchini with golden potatoes 69
24. Chicken Wings and Ham, with Chimichurri 70
25. Goat cheese salad 71
26. Pilar House Eggs 71
27. potato balls 72
28. Harness Croquettes 73
29. Uncle Pepe croquettes 74
30. Baked york cheese, egg and ham potatoes 75
31. Salmon in a bread crumb 75
32. Kassler Sauerkraut Balls 76
33. Sweet sweets from the airfryer 77
34. Green Shakshuka with the Airfryer baking pan 78
35. Avocado on toast with poached egg! 78
36. A BREAD ROLL AND AN EGG 79
37. Cordon Bleu Balls 80
38. Cheese ham pluck bread 81
39. Green focaccia from the Philips Airfryer 82
40. chicken tikka masala 82
41. Persian herbal frittata 83

42. Fried halloumi with asparagus salad 84
43. Juicy Lemon Ricotta Cake with the Airfryer 85
44. French Onion Soup Grilled Cheese Sandwich 86
45. Bananas marble cake with the baking dish 87
46. Apple chips from the airfryer 88
47. Vegetable chips with the snack kit 88
48. Three quiche in the Airfryer baking pan 89
49. Stuffed Mediterranean peppers with the party kit 92
50. Pizza Flammkuchen Style from the Airfryer 92
51. Beef and Onion BBQ Pizza from the Airfryer 94
52. Cheese sticks from the Philips Airfryer 94
53. Baltic Garlic Bread Sticks With Yogurt Dip 95
54. Muzen from the Airfryer 96
55. Roasted almonds from the airfryer 97
56. Avocado fries from the airfryer 97
57 Banana Bread Waffles with the Philips Airfryer 98
58. Raclette in the airfryer 98
59 Stuffed mushrooms from the airfryer 100
60. Hot chestnuts from the airfryer 100
61. Burnt almonds from the airfryer 101
62 Wine pears in dressing gown 101
63 Roast beef with potato gratin and Bernaise sauce 102
64 Goat cheese tartlets with figs, salad & pistachios 103
65 Baked apple from the airfryer 104
66 Rack of lamb with herb crust from the airfryer 105
67 Spicy carrots from the airfryer 106
68 Beetroot carpaccio with pistachio crisp 107
69 Panettone from the Airfryer 108
70 Coq au vin from the airfryer 109
71 Baked gorgonzola pears from the airfryer 110
72 Balsamic Brussels sprouts from the airfryer 111
73 Eggplant salad from the airfryer 112
74 Nutty goat's cheese from the airfryer 112
75 Perfect donuts from the airfryer 114
76 Three-grain bread from the Airfryer baking pan 115
77 Fish in sesame crust from the airfryer 116
78 Berry Crumble from the Airfryer 117
79 Fluffy pancakes from the Airfryer baking dish 118
80 Beef roulades from the airfryer 119
81 Eggplant chips from the Philips Airfryer 119
82 Potato wedges from the Philips Airfryer 120
83 Cordon Bleu from the Philips Airfryer 120
84 Camembert in the loaf of bread from the Philips Airfryer 121
85 Sweet potato fritters from the Philips Airfryer 122
86 Zucchini fries with peanut breading 123
87 Vitelotte fries from the Philips Airfryer 123
88 Halloween snack from the Philips Airfryer 124

89	Warm pumpkin salad with cashew nuts and goat cheese	124
90	Original apple strudel from the Philips Airfryer	125
91	Sweet potato slices with salsa from the airfryer	126
92	Orange chicken fillets from the Philips Airfryer	127
93	Bun Thit Nuong	128
94	Party shrimp skewers from the airfryer	130
95	Filled burger from the airfryer	131
96	Our absolute favorite waffle recipe!	132
97	Galette from the airfryer	133
98	Mediterranean aubergine with Tahini dressing	134
99	Crispy sushi	135
100	Stuffed tomatoes from the Philips Airfryer	137
101	Sweet bacon muffins with maple syrup	138
102	Apple rings - a round thing	139
103	Salmon with fennel and orange from the airfryer	140
104	Tornado potatoes with bacon and cheese from the airfryer	141
105	Poached eggs from the airfryer	141
106	Burger dumplings from the Airfryer: crazy and damn delicious	142
107	Cheese volcano from the Airfryer - the sociable snack	143
108	Samosas - Crunchy, Spicy, Tasty	144
109	Tornado potatoes with bacon and onions	146
110	Broccoli croquettes	146
111	English breakfast	147
112	Frikandeln Speciaal - Dutch meat rolls with mayo and onions	148

Part 1

Chapter 1: Introduction

If you're reading this book now, then you've either bought an air fryer already and are looking for recipes to use with it, or you're thinking about buying one and want more information on what you can make with it. Either way, this book is great for you and I am glad you're giving it a chance! First, I'm going to give you an introduction to what an air fryer is, how it works and its benefits and advantages. I realize this is a bit tedious for those of you who already own one, and if you prefer, you can just jump straight to the recipes and start baking up some yummy desserts, starting in chapter 2! But for those who are new to the idea…

What is an air fryer, and how does it work?

It's quite simple. An air fryer is an appliance that fries up food using hot air, which circulates at a high speed around the food inside it. This is different from a deep fryer, which fries using oil. While an air fryer does use oil, too, it only uses around a tablespoon or less to work its magic.

What are the benefits and advantages to using an air fryer?

First, let me start with the health benefits and advantages to cooking with an air fryer versus cooking with a deep fryer:

- Deep fryers typically fry away the good nutrients from food. Air fryers keep the nutrients in while still providing the fried goodness you love.
- Because deep fryers use a huge amount of oil, there are times when the oil can add bad fats to your food, which can then lead to bad problems with your body, such as a higher risk of cancer, obesity, heart disease and kidney disease.

Secondly, the other benefits:

- It's great for people like busy moms, college students, and more, because you can just let the food cook while you're off doing house chores, studying, or whatever you need to do while you wait.
- It's not just for fried foods; it's also for baking! You will find that there are many recipes in here for items you would think could only be done in an oven, such as cakes, cupcakes, and even cookies.
- It's easy and simple to use, by just putting in the food and doing a couple of button presses.
- It's safe to use, because most come with an automatic shutdown feature, so if you're so busy you aren't paying attention to the timer, be assured that the air fryer won't keep cooking and burn your food or worse. Not only that, but because you are only using a minimal amount of oil and the air fryer is closed while cooking, there is no risk of injury from hot oil splattering out.

- You have many appliances all in one, because an air fryer can bake, roast and grill, thereby saving you from having to have a deep fryer, toaster, oven, skillet, or grill. Therefore you also save counter space in your kitchen by only having to have one appliance that is also compact.
- It's easy to clean in that the removable parts, such as the basket that comes with the air fryer, can be safely put into a dishwasher. If you don't have a dishwasher, however, it's still an easy job by just soaking the parts for a bit and then using a clean sponge to gently rub out the food bits that are stuck to the air fryer parts.
- You save money on all that cooking oil you're not using for a deep fryer.
- Additionally to saving money on cooking oil, when cooking with it, oil vapors deposit onto your counter tops, walls and floors. By using an air fryer, you won't have that problem.

Chapter 2: Breakfast Sweets

Cinnamon and Sugar Donuts

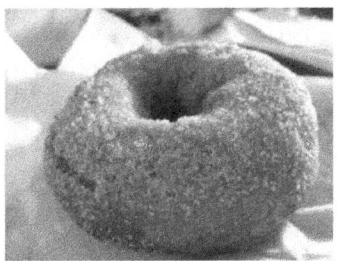

Yield: 9 servings

Time to make: about 35 minutes

Ingredients:

For the Donuts:

- 2 tablespoons of butter at room temperature + 1/3 cup of butter, melted - separated
- 1/2 cup of sugar
- 2 1/4 cups of plain flour
- 1 1/2 teaspoons of baking powder
- 1 teaspoon of salt
- 2 large egg yolks

- 1/2 cup of sour cream
- 1/3 cup of butter, melted

For the Cinnamon Sugar Coating:

- 1/3 cup of caster sugar
- 1 teaspoon of cinnamon

Directions:

1. Using clean hands and in a bowl, press together the room temperature butter and the sugar until it is all crumbly. Then stir in the egg yolks until it is well-combined.
2. Put the flour, baking powder, and salt in a sifter or fine-meshed strainer or sieve, and then sift it into another bowl.
3. Then add 1/3 of the flour mix plus 1/2 of the sour cream into another bowl. Stir until well combined before adding another 1/3 of the flour mix and 1/2 of the sour cream. Mix again. Then place the mixture into the fridge for a bit.
4. Make the cinnamon sugar mixture by mixing together the cinnamon and sugar in a bowl large enough to dip the donuts into (or a plate).
5. Lightly flour your work surface and then roll out the dough until it is about a centimeter thick. Now you have several ways to cut out the donuts. You can use a donut cutter, if you have one, or use a large circle cookie cutter to cut out the donut followed by a small circle cookie cutter to cut out the center.
6. Preheat the air fryer to 350 degrees F/180 degrees C.
7. Brush both sides of each donut with some melted butter, and then add it to the air fryer to fry for about 8 minutes.
8. When done, immediately brush again with more melted butter and then dip both sides of the donuts into the cinnamon sugar mixture.
9. Serve warm or cold.

Note: The donut holes can be made into cinnamon sugar donut holes by adding them to the air fryer, too.

Blueberry Muffins

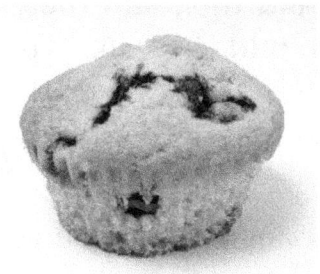

Yield: 10 to 11 small muffins

Time to make: about 30 minutes

Ingredients:
- 1/2 cup of cake flour or regular flour
- 1/2 cup or less (depending on desired sweetness) of sugar
- 1/2 teaspoon of salt
- 2 teaspoons of baking powder
- 1/3 cup of vegetable oil
- 1 egg
- up to 1 cup of yogurt
- 2 teaspoons of vanilla extract
- 1 cup of blueberries, washed and drained

Directions:
1. With the blueberries in a large bowl, coat them thoroughly with the flour.
2. In a separate bowl, combine the flour, sugar, salt and baking powder. Then whisk it to make sure the salt and baking powder is spread evenly.
3. Put the oil in a measuring cup, and then add the egg. Start adding the yogurt until you have one full cup. Then add the vanilla extract and stir with a whisk until it is fully combined.
4. Using a fork, combine the wet ingredients with the dry ingredients, but do not overmix.
5. Next, gently fold in the blueberries with a spoon or spatula.
6. Remove the air fryer basket, and preheat the air fryer to 350 degrees F/180 degrees C and let it preheat for 10 minutes.
7. With the blueberries in a large bowl, coat them thoroughly with the flour.

8. In a separate bowl, combine the flour, sugar, salt and baking powder. Then whisk it to make sure the salt and baking powder is spread evenly.
9. Put the oil in a measuring cup, and then add the egg. Start adding the yogurt until you have one full cup. Then add the vanilla extract and stir with a whisk until it is fully combined.
10. Using a fork, combine the wet ingredients with the dry ingredients, but do not overmix.
11. Next, gently fold in the blueberries with a spoon or spatula.
12. Remove the air fryer basket, and preheat the air fryer to 350 degrees F/180 degrees C and let it preheat for 10 minutes.
13. Meanwhile, place 4 or 5 muffins cups (whatever you can fit) into the basket of the air fryer. Fill each cup to about 3/4 full of the muffin batter. Finally, sprinkle some brown sugar onto the top of each muffin.
14. Bake for 10 minutes at 350 degrees F/180 degrees F, then check if they are done by inserting a toothpick in and seeing if it comes out clean. If any are not done at this point, they can be baked for a couple of more minutes and then checked again. (Leave out the ones that are done.)
15. Repeat with the remaining batter.

Double the Chocolate Muffins

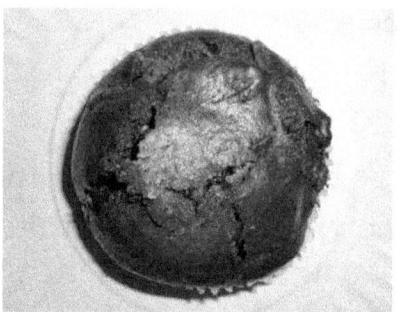

Yield: 12 muffins

Time to make: about 45 minutes

Ingredients:
- 2 1/2 cups of self-rising flour
- 1 cup of brown sugar

- 1/3 cup of unsweetened cocoa powder
- 6 ounces of semi-sweet chocolate chips
- 2 eggs
- 1 cup of milk
- 2/3 cup of butter, melted, or 2/3 cup of vegetable oil

Directions:

1. Preheat the air fryer to 350 degrees F/160 degrees F.
2. Combine together the flour, brown sugar, cocoa powder and chocolate chips into a bowl and mix well with a whisk.
3. Whisk together the eggs, milk and melted butter in a separate bowl until it is smooth and well-combined.
4. Add the dry mixture to the wet, and then stir with a spoon or spatula until it is just combined but not overmixed.
5. Fill 6 silicone muffin cups or regular paper muffin cups to about 3/4 full with the muffin batter and place in the air fryer. You can bake more if your air fryer can fit more.
6. Bake for 13 to 15 minutes, until it is firm to the touch and a toothpick inserted comes out clean.
7. Repeat process for the remaining 6 muffins.

Cinnamon or Vanilla French Toast Sticks

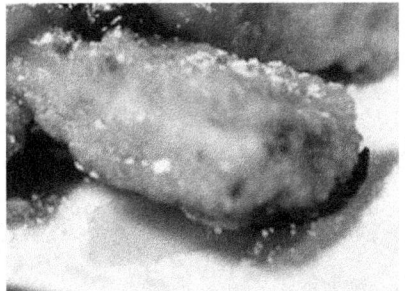

Yield: 2 servings

Time to make: about 20 minutes

Ingredients:
- 4 pieces of sliced bread of choice, any thickness
- about 2 tablespoons or so of soft butter or margarine

- 2 eggs, gently beaten
- a sprinkle of salt
- cinnamon, to taste, or vanilla extract, to taste
- maple syrup, for serving
- cooking spray

Directions:

1. Preheat the air fryer to 350 degrees F/180 degrees C.
2. Place the gently beaten eggs in a bowl and mix in the salt and the cinnamon or vanilla (a teaspoon or two should be enough).
3. Butter both sides of the slices of bread. Then cut into 4 to 6 strips per slice.
4. Dip the buttered bread sticks into the egg mixture, making sure to cover both sides and drench them well. Arrange them in the air fryer as you go along. You will need to do this in two batches.
5. For the first batch, cook for 2 minutes. Then pause the air fryer, remove the pan to a heat-safe surface, and spray the bread sticks with some cooking spray generously.
6. Carefully flip them over to generously spray the other side and return the pan to the air fryer to cook for another 4 minutes, checking after 2 minutes to make sure they are cooking evenly and haven't burnt.
7. Remove when the egg on the bread sticks is cooked and the bread sticks themselves are golden brown in color. Transfer them to a plate and then follow the same process for the second batch (steps 5 and 6).
8. Serve with the maple syrup for dipping, or drizzle the maple syrup on top of the sticks.

Plain Donuts With Strawberry Icing

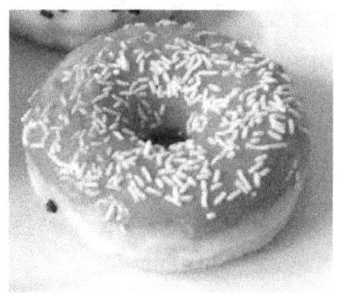

Yield: 4 servings

Time to make: 25 minutes

Ingredients:
- 1 1/2 cups of self-rising flour
- 1/3 cup of caster sugar
- 1/3 cup of brown sugar
- 1/2 cup of whole milk
- 1 teaspoon of baking powder
- 2 1/2 tablespoons of butter
- 1 large egg
- strawberry icing (or alternatively you can use chocolate, vanilla...whatever you fancy)
- sprinkles, for decoration, if desired

Directions:
1. Preheat the air fryer to 350 degrees F/180 degrees C.
2. Put the flour in a medium mixing bowl.
3. Mix together the milk, butter and egg in a separate mixing bowl.
4. Then add the milk-butter-egg mixture to the flour and then mix until it is just combined, but do not overmix.
5. Use a donut cutter or two separate round cutters to make four donut shapes.
6. Grease an air fryer baking pan and then arrange the donuts onto it. Cook for 15 minutes, until they spring back when you lightly press them.
7. Remove and let cool for 5 minutes before spreading on your favorite icing. Then add sprinkles if desired.

Chocolate Eclairs

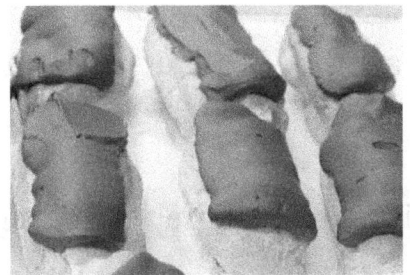

Yield: 9 servings

Time to make: 40 minutes

Ingredients:

For the Éclair Dough:

- 1/4 cup of butter
- 3/4 cup of flour
- 3 medium eggs
- 2/3 cup of water

For the Filling:

- 1 teaspoon of vanilla essence
- 1 teaspoon of icing sugar
- 3/4 cup of whipped cream

Chocolate Topping:

- 2 ounces of milk chocolate, chopped into chunks
- 1 tablespoon of whipped cream
- 1/8 cup of butter

Directions:

For the Éclair Dough:

1. Preheat the air fryer to 350 degrees F/180 degrees C.
2. Meanwhile, in a large pan, place the butter into the water and melt it over medium heat. Then bring it to a boil. Remove from heat.
3. Stir in the flour.
4. Return the pan to the heat, and stir it until a medium ball of dough forms in the middle of the pan. Remove from heat and transfer the dough to a bowl to let cool.
5. Once cooled, beat in the eggs until you have a smooth mixture of dough.
6. Divide it up into 9 éclair-shaped dough pieces, and then add them to the air fryer to bake for 10 minutes. Then reduce heat to 325 degrees F/160 degrees F and continue to bake for another 8 minutes. Meanwhile, you can work on the filling as follows.

For the Filling:

7. In a bowl and using a whisk, mix together the filling ingredients until you get a nice, thick mixture.
8. When the éclairs are ready, take them out to cool and make the chocolate topping as follows…

For the Chocolate Topping:

9. Put the chocolate topping ingredients into a glass bowl and place it over a pan of hot water. Mix until the chocolate melts.
10. When the éclairs are nice and cool, top them with the melted chocolate.

Breakfast or Tea Time Scones

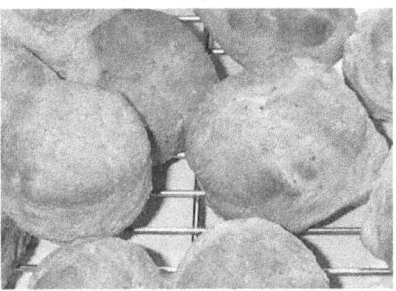

Yield: 4 servings

Time to make: 15 to 25 minutes

Ingredients:
- 2 cups of self-rising flour, sifted
- 1/2 teaspoon of salt
- 1 teaspoon of sugar
- 1 tablespoon of butter
- 3/4 cup of milk
- your favorite jam, for serving

Directions:
1. Preheat the air fryer to 375 degrees F/190 degrees C.
2. In a bowl, stir the flour together with the salt and sugar.
3. Using clean hands, rub in the butter into the flour, salt and sugar mix until you get something that resembles breadcrumbs.
4. Use your fingers to make a hole in center of the flour. Then pour the milk into the center.
5. Mix it all together lightly but also quickly to get a dough for the scones.
6. Flour your work surface, and transfer the dough to it, and then knead the dough lightly.
7. Pat it out until you get a 1/4-inch thickness of dough.
8. Take a 2-inch-round cutter and dip it into some flour. Then cut the dough into scone-shaped rounds, making sure to dip the cutter in between cuts each time.

9. Lightly grease the baking tray of the air fryer and brush each of the tops of the scones with a little milk.
10. Bake in the air fryer for 10 minutes, until they are golden brown.
11. Serve with your favorite jam.

Chapter 3: Cookies And Brownies

Chocolate Brownies

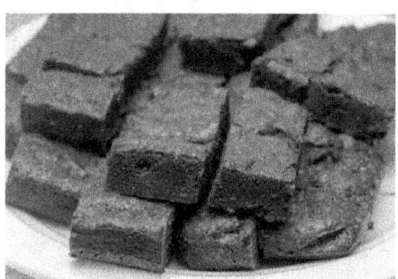

Yield: 4 servings

Time to make: 20 minutes

Ingredients:
- 1/2 cup of butter
- 2 ounces of chocolate
- 1 cup of brown sugar
- 2 medium eggs, beaten
- 2 teaspoons of vanilla essence
- 3/4 cup of self-rising flour

Directions:
1. Preheat the air fryer to 350 degrees F/180 degrees C.
2. Place the chocolate and butter in a medium bowl and then place the bowl over a pan of hot water until the chocolate melts.
3. Once melted, take it off heat and stir in the brown sugar, followed by the beaten eggs, and then the vanilla essence. Finally, add the self-rising flour and mix it well.
4. Transfer the resulting brownie batter into a pan that fits into your air fryer. (You may have to do more than one batch.) Bake for 15 minutes in the preheated air fryer.

5. When they are done, let them cool for a little bit before cutting them into squares to serve.

Note: If you'd like to add some walnuts, stir in about 1/3 cup as the final ingredient before putting them in the air fryer.

Oatmeal Raisin Cookies

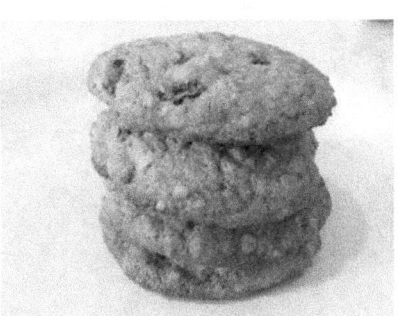

Yield: 1 dozen or more cookies, depending on size made

Time to make: 15 minutes

Ingredients:
- 1 1/2 cups oats, ground
- 3/4 cup of cashews, ground
- 2 teaspoons of cinnamon
- 1 1/2 teaspoon of vanilla extract
- 1 teaspoon of baking powder
- a pinch of salt
- 2 tablespoons of ground flaxseeds, soaked in a 1/2-cup of water
- 1 cup of sugar
- 3/4 cup of raisins

Directions:
1. Preheat the air fryer to 350 degrees F/180 degrees C.
2. Combine the oats, cashews, cinnamon, baking powder and salt in a bowl and mix well.
3. Then add the vanilla, sugar and flaxseed with the water and mix well again.
4. Finally, add the raisins and give it another stir. Add more water, if necessary, to make a dough that is sticky.

5. Divide the dough up and roll it into balls. Then flatten each ball a little.
6. Transfer them to the wire basket of the air fryer, and then bake for 8 minutes.
7. When done, let cool completely before serving.

Chocolate Chip Cookies

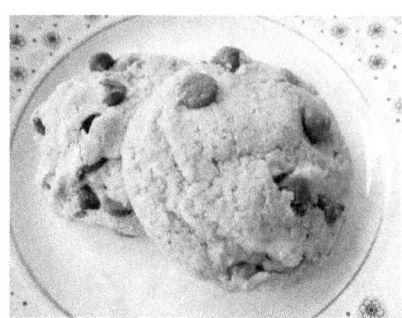

Yield: 9 cookies or more, depending on size made

Time to make: about 15 minutes

Ingredients:
- 1/2 cup of butter
- 1/2 cup of brown sugar
- 1 1/4 cups of self-rising flour
- 1 cup of semisweet chocolate chips
- 2 tablespoons of honey
- 1 tablespoon of milk

Directions:
1. Preheat the air fryer to 350 degrees F/180 degrees C.
2. Beat the butter in a large mixing bowl until it is soft. Then add the sugar and combine until the mixture is light and fluffy.
3. Next, stir in the honey and flour. Mix well.
4. Then stir in the chocolate chips.
5. Finally, add the milk and stir it well.
6. Spoon the dough onto an air-fryer-sized cookie sheet and bake for 6 minutes before reducing the temperature to 325 degrees F/160 degrees F to bake for another 2 minutes to complete baking. If doing this in batches, you will need to repeat this for each batch.
7. Serve nice and warm.

Peanut Butter Cookies

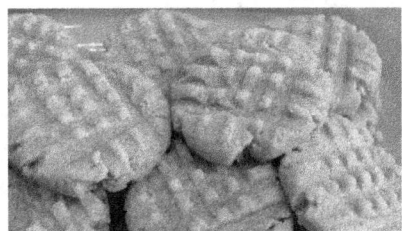

Yield: 1 to 2 dozen, depending on size made

Time to make: 30 minutes or more, depending on number of batches, plus chill time

Ingredients:
- 1/2 cup of butter, at room temperature
- 1/2 cup of sugar
- 1/2 cup of packed brown sugar
- 1/2 cup of peanut butter
- 1 egg
- 1 1/2 cups of all-purpose flour
- 3/4 teaspoon of baking soda
- 1/2 teaspoon of baking powder
- 1/4 teaspoon of salt

Directions:
1. In a bowl, beat the butter for 2 minutes, until it is creamy. Then add the sugar to the butter and mix for another 2 minutes. Next, add the peanut butter and the egg.
2. In a separate bowl, whisk up the flour, baking soda, baking powder, and the salt, vigorously.
3. Mix the dry ingredient mix in with the sugar – butter mixture.
4. Transfer the resulting dough into a piece of plastic, wrap it up, and place in the fridge for at least 3 hours.
5. Later on, preheat the air fryer to 350 degrees F/180 degrees C. Shape the dough into balls and lay them out 3 inches apart on an air-fryer-sized baking sheet. You will need to do this in batches. Using a fork, flatten the balls and also make a crisscross pattern across them.

6. Place in the air fryer to bake for 8 to 10 minutes, until they are a light brown color. Repeat as necessary until all the batches are done.
7. Remove and let cool for a bit before serving.

Snickerdoodles

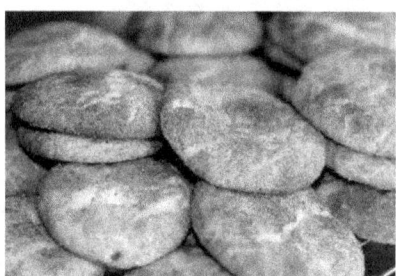

Yield: 2 dozen

Time to make: about 1 hour

Ingredients:
- 1 cup of butter
- 1 1/2 cups of sugar + 3 tablespoons of sugar, separated
- 2 large eggs
- 2 3/4 cups flour
- 2 teaspoons of cream of tartar
- 1 teaspoon of baking soda
- 1/4 teaspoon of salt
- 3 teaspoons of cinnamon

Directions:
1. In a large mixing bowl, thoroughly mix together the butter, the 1 1/2 cups of sugar and eggs.
2. Then, in another bowl, combine together the flour, cream of tartar, baking soda and salt.
3. Blend the two mixtures together in another bowl from dry mixture to butter mixture.
4. Transfer the dough to a piece of plastic wrap, wrap it up and chill in the fridge, along with an air-fryer-size baking sheet.
5. In the meantime, in a small bowl, mix together the remaining sugar with 3 tablespoons of the cinnamon.

6. Preheat the air fryer to 350 degrees F/180 degrees C.
7. Once chilled, roll the dough into 1-inch balls and then dip each ball into the cinnamon sugar mixture before placing them on the chilled baking sheet. You will need to do more than one batch, so chill the baking sheet each time (or chill several at once).
8. Bake each batch in the preheated air fryer for about 8 to 10 minutes, until they are a nice, light brown color.

Cheesecake Swirl Brownies

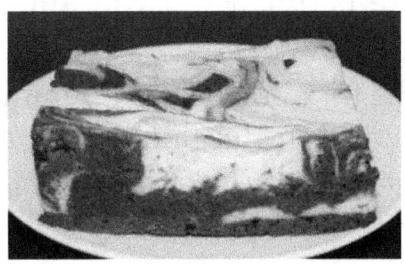

Yield: 4 servings

Time to make: 25 to 30 minutes

Ingredients:

For the Brownie:

- 1/2 cup of butter
- 2 ounces of chocolate
- 1 cup of brown sugar
- 2 medium eggs, beaten
- 2 teaspoons of vanilla essence
- 3/4 cup of self-rising flour

For the Cheesecake:

- 3 ounces of cream cheese, at room temperature
- 1/4 cup of sour cream
- 2 tablespoons of icing sugar

Directions:

For the Brownie:

1. Preheat the air fryer to 350 degrees F/180 degrees C.

2. Place the chocolate and butter in a medium bowl and then place the bowl over a pan of hot water until the chocolate melts.
3. Once melted, take it off heat and stir in the brown sugar, followed by the beaten eggs, and then the vanilla essence. Finally, add the self-rising flour and mix it well.
4. Transfer the resulting brownie batter into a pan that fits into your air fryer. Set aside while you make the cheesecake.

For the Cheesecake:

5. In a medium bowl and using an electric mixer, beat all of the cheesecake ingredients together until smooth.
6. Drop dollops of cheesecake batter across the top of the brownie batter, then make swirls with a knife.
7. Place in the air fryer to bake for about 15 to 20 minutes, and then check to see if a toothpick or skewer inserted in the middle comes out with a few lumps but not totally clean. If not, continue to bake a little bit longer, checking every few minutes.
8. Let cool before cutting and serving.

Mint Chocolate Brownies

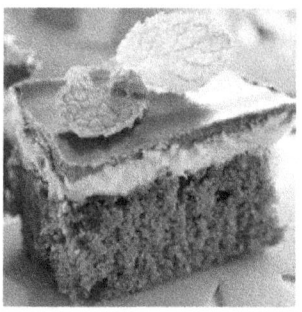

Yield: 4 servings

Time to make: 45 minutes plus time to chill

Ingredients:

For the Brownie Layer:

- 1/2 cup of butter
- 2 ounces of chocolate
- 1 cup of brown sugar
- 2 medium eggs, beaten

- 2 teaspoons of vanilla essence
- 3/4 cup of self-rising flour

For the Mint Layer:

- 1/4 cup of unsalted butter, softened and at room temperature
- 1 cup of confectioner's sugar
- 1 tablespoon of milk
- 3/4 teaspoon of peppermint extract
- 1 drop of liquid or gel green food coloring, if desired

For the Chocolate Layer:

- 1/4 cup of unsalted butter
- 1/2 cup of semisweet chocolate chips

Directions:

For the Brownie Layer:

1. Preheat the air fryer to 350 degrees F/180 degrees C.
2. Place the chocolate and butter in a medium bowl and then place the bowl over a pan of hot water until the chocolate melts.
3. Once melted, take it off heat and stir in the brown sugar, followed by the beaten eggs, and then the vanilla essence. Finally, add the self-rising flour and mix it well.
4. Transfer the resulting brownie batter into a pan that fits into your air fryer. Bake for 15 minutes in the preheated air fryer.
5. Once done, let cool and then transfer to a baking sheet in preparation for the next two layers as follows.

For the Mint Layer:

6. Beat the butter in a medium bowl using a handheld or stand mixer until the butter is smooth and creamy, around 2 minutes.
7. Then add the confectioners' sugar and the milk and beat for another 2 minutes on low speed. Increase to high speed and beat for another minute.
8. Next, add the peppermint extract and, if using, the green food coloring. Beat on high speed for another minute.
9. Give it a taste, and add more peppermint if needed
10. Layer it onto the top of the brownie layer, and then place in the fridge to set for 1 to 4 hours.

For the Chocolate Layer (after the 1 to 4 hours set time):

11. Place the chocolate and butter in a medium bowl and then place the bowl over a pan of hot water until the chocolate melts.
12. Spread this across the mint layer using a knife or spatula, and then put back in the fridge to set once again for 1 to 4 hours.
13. Once done, use a very sharp large knife to slice them into squares.

Chapter 4: Cakes And Cupcakes

Red Velvet Cupcakes

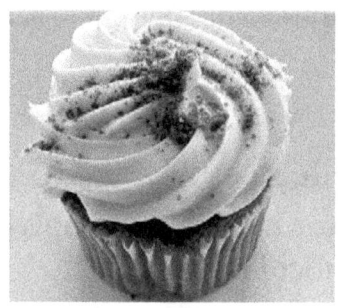

Yield: 20 servings

Time to make: about 1 hour

Ingredients:
- 1/2 cup of butter
- 1 1/2 cups white sugar
- 2 eggs
- 1 cup of buttermilk
- 1 ounce of red food coloring
- 1 teaspoon of vanilla extract
- 1 1/2 teaspoons of baking soda
- 1 tablespoon of distilled white vinegar
- 2 cups of all-purpose flour
- 1/3 cup of unsweetened cocoa powder
- 1 teaspoon of salt
- 1 to 2 containers of frosting of choice
- red sprinkles or other decoration of choice, if desired

Directions:
1. Preheat the air fryer to 350 degrees F/180 degrees F.
2. Beat the butter and sugar together in a large bowl, using an electric mixer, until the mixture is light and fluffy. Then mix in the eggs, buttermilk, red food coloring and the vanilla. Next, stir in the baking soda and the vinegar.
3. In a separate bowl, combine the flour, cocoa powder and salt together and then stir that into the mix with the rest of the ingredients from step 2 until just blended.
4. Fill silicone baking cups with about 2/3 full with batter. You will need to bake the cupcakes in batches.
5. Cook the first batch at 350 degrees F/180 degrees F for 5 minutes, and then reduce heat to 340 degrees F/170 degrees F for 10 to 12 minutes. Repeat this baking process with all the batches.
6. Set the cupcakes aside to cool before frosting them with your favorite frosting and sprinkling your favorite decoration on top.

Dreamy Chocolate Cake

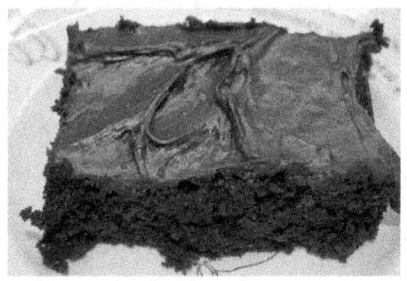

Yield: 8 servings

Time to make: about 1 hour

Ingredients:
- 1 cup of brown sugar
- 3/4 cup of all-purpose flour
- 1/2 cup of unsweetened cocoa powder
- 3/4 teaspoon of baking powder
- 3/4 teaspoon of baking soda
- 1/2 teaspoon of salt

- 1 large egg
- 1/2 cup of milk
- 1/4 cup of vegetable oil
- 1 teaspoon of vanilla extract
- 1/2 cup of hot water
- optional: 1 teaspoon of instant coffee mix for more flavor, your favorite frosting or icing

Directions:

1. Preheat the air fryer to 350 degrees F/180 degrees C for 5 minutes.
2. Stir together the sugar, flour, cocoa powder, baking powder, baking soda and salt in a large mixing bowl.
3. Then add the egg, milk, oil and vanilla extract, and gently stir until it is evenly mixed.
4. If using instant coffee mix, mix it into the hot water and then stir it into the mixture. If not, then just the hot water alone. Mix until it is evenly mixed. Batter is okay if it looks to be thinning.
5. Transfer the mixture to the air fryer baking pan and cover with foil. Then poke some random holes into the foil.
6. Reduce temperature to 325 degrees F/160 degrees F, and then bake the cake in the air fryer for 35 minutes.
7. Remove the foil, keeping the temperature the same, and bake for an additional 10 minutes, until a skewer inserted into the cake comes out clean.
8. Let cool for 10 minutes before cutting and serving.
9. Frost with your favorite frosting or icing if desired, or eat plain.

Marvelous Marble Cake

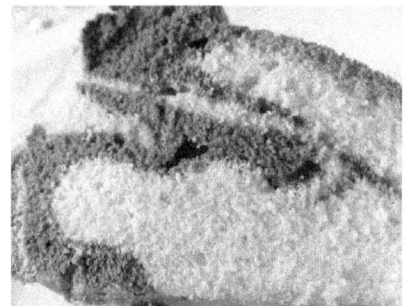

Yield: 6 to 8 servings

Time to make: about 25 minutes

Ingredients:
- 2/3 cup of butter, melted
- 1/2 cup of sugar
- 3 large eggs, beaten
- 1 tablespoon of cocoa powder
- 3/4 cup of self-rising flour, sifted
- 1/2 teaspoon of lemon juice

Directions:
1. Preheat the air fryer to 350 degrees F/180 degrees F. Grease an air fryer baking pan and set aside while you prepare the batter.
2. Put about 1/3 of the melted butter in a bowl and mix in the cocoa powder until you have a smooth paste. Set aside. This will be the cocoa mixture.
3. In a separate bowl, beat the remaining melted butter with the sugar until it is pale.
4. Add the eggs to the butter mixture from step 3 and then alternate it with the flour, beating until smooth. Then add the lemon juice and mix well. This will be the plain cake mixture.
5. Transfer the plain cake mixture into the air fryer baking pan while alternating with the cocoa mixture. Use a knife to create swirls when done.
6. Place in the air fryer to bake for about 15 to 17 minutes until it is completely baked and a skewer inserted into it comes out clean.
7. Let cool in the pan and then remove to a cooling rack to continue to cool before serving.

Amazing Molten Lava Cake

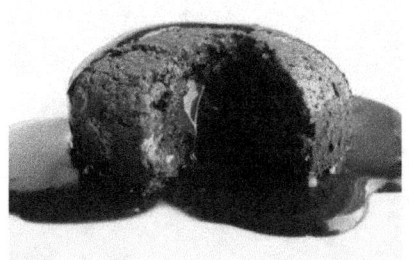

Yield: 4 servings

Time to make: 20 minutes

Ingredients:
- 4 ounces of dark chocolate, chopped
- 1/2 cup of butter
- 1/2 orange, juiced
- 2 eggs
- 1/2 cup of brown sugar
- 1/2 teaspoon instant coffee
- 1/2 cup of flour
- 1/4 tablespoon of baking powder
- a pinch of salt
- butter, for greasing the baking pan

Directions:
1. Place the chocolate and butter in a medium bowl and then place the bowl over a pan of hot water until the chocolate slowly melts. Then remove from heat and add in the orange juice. Stir well to combine.
2. Mix the eggs with the sugar and instant coffee in a separate bowl. Then use an electric mixer to beat it until creamy. Once creamy, stir in the chocolate orange mixture.
3. Next, mix in the flour, baking powder and the salt, but only until it is slightly mixed.
4. Preheat the air fryer to 350 degrees F/180 degrees C. Butter the air fryer baking pan.
5. Pour the batter into the prepared baking pan and bake for 10 minutes. Cake is done when it is firm to the touch.

Carrot Cake with Cream Cheese Frosting

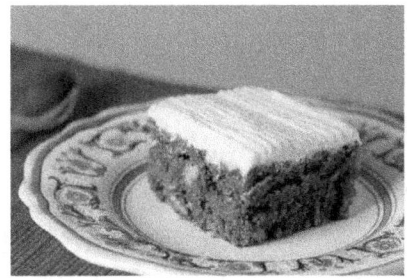

Yield: 12 to 16 servings/2 six-inch cakes

Time to make: about 45 minutes

Ingredients:

For the Carrot Cake:

- 2 cups of all-purpose flour
- 2 teaspoons of baking soda
- 1/2 teaspoon of salt
- 1 1/2 teaspoon of cinnamon
- 3 eggs, at room temperature
- 1/3 cup of sugar
- 1/4 cup of honey
- 2/3 cup of sunflower oil
- 2 teaspoons of vanilla essence
- 1/2 cup of applesauce
- 1/4 cup of plain yogurt
- 2 1/2 cups of carrots, shredded
- 1/2 cup of walnuts

For the Cream Cheese Frosting:

- 8 ounces of cream cheese
- 1 cup of icing sugar
- 1/2 cup of plain yogurt
- 1 teaspoon of vanilla essence
- 1 tablespoon of lemon juice, if desired, to make it more tangy

Note: you will need to make the cream cheese ahead of time to make sure it is thickened enough to frost the cake with. See instructions below.

Directions:

For the Cream Cheese Frosting:

1. Beat the cream cheese until it is softened.
2. A little at a time, add the icing sugar and mix until it is not visible.
3. Then repeat the same process with the yogurt.
4. Add the vanilla and lemon juice. Beat it again until the frosting is completely smooth.
5. Transfer to a container, cover, and chill in the fridge for a couple of hours before using it to frost the carrot cake.

For the Carrot Cake:

6. Grease the baking pan and line the bottom of it with parchment paper.
7. Sift together the all-purpose flour, baking soda, cinnamon and salt into a medium-sized bowl, and then set aside.
8. With a handheld mixer on medium speed, combine the sugar and oil in a large bowl. Then mix in the yogurt and applesauce for about 1 minute, until fully combined.
9. Next, beat in the eggs, one at a time.
10. Then mix in the vanilla.
11. Preheat the air fryer to 347 degrees F/175 degrees C.
12. Using a spatula, stir the wet ingredients into the dry until just combined and all of the flour pockets are gone, but do not overmix.
13. Finally, stir in the carrots and walnuts.
14. Pour into the air fryer baking pan and then bake it for 30 minutes.
15. Remove and let cool before frosting with the cream cheese.

Happy Birthday Cake

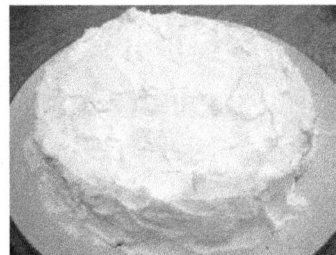

Note that this wonderfully yummy cake can really be used for any occasion.

Yield: 8 to 10 servings

Time to make: about 1 hour

Ingredients:
- 2 1/2 cups of all-purpose flour, sifted
- 1 1/4 cups of sugar
- 3 eggs
- 3 teaspoons of baking powder
- 1/4 teaspoon of salt
- 3/4 cup of butter, softened
- 1 cup of milk
- 1 teaspoon of vanilla
- white frosting or any other flavor of choice

Directions:
1. Preheat the air fryer for 3 minutes at 325 degrees F/160 degrees F.
2. Butter or spray with nonstick oil the bottoms of two air fryer baking pans.
3. In a bowl, combine the sifted flour, baking powder and the salt.
4. In another bowl, use an electric mixer to beat together the sugar with the butter.
5. Then, add the eggs and the vanilla to the sugar-butter mixture. Beat until it is mixed fully.
6. Add the flour mixture alternately with the milk to the sugar-butter mixture. Beat well each time until it is mixed fully.
7. Divide the cake batter between the two cake pans.
8. Then bake each pan in the air fryer for 20 to 24 minutes, until a toothpick or skewer inserted into the center comes out clean.

9. Let them both cool on wire racks before assembling the cake by frosting the top of one layer, placing the second layer on top, and then frosting all around.

For the Cream Cheese Frosting:

10. Beat the cream cheese until it is softened.
11. A little at a time, add the icing sugar and mix until it is not visible.
12. Then repeat the same process with the yogurt.
13. Add the vanilla and lemon juice. Beat it again until the frosting is completely smooth.

Vanilla Chiffon Cake

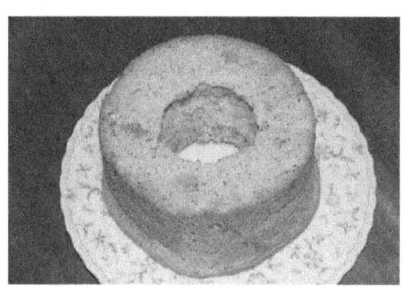

Yield: 6 to 8 servings

Time to make: about 45 minutes

Ingredients:
- 1 1/2 ounces of cake flour or plain flour, sifted
- 1/4 teaspoon of baking powder, sifted
- 2 egg yolks
- 2 egg whites
- 1/2 ounce + 1 ounce of castor sugar, separated
- 1 teaspoon of vanilla extract
- 2 1/3 tablespoons of vegetable oil
- 1/4 cup of milk
- 1/8 teaspoon of cream of tartar

Directions:
1. Place the egg yolks, 1/2 ounce of castor sugar, vanilla extract, vegetable oil and milk in a mixing bowl, and then, using a hand whisk, beat until it is combined and the sugar is dissolved.

2. Then add the flour, and whisk again until it is well combined. Set aside.
3. In a separate bowl, beat the egg whites, the 1 ounce of castor sugar and the cream of tartar for about 5 minutes with a hand mixer until you have stiff peaks forming. This is the meringue for the cake.
4. Remove about 1/3 of the meringue and, using a hand whisk, mix it into the yolk mixture.
5. Repeat again with 1/3 of the meringue at a time, and whisk each time until you have no white streaks left in the resulting cake batter.
6. Preheat the air fryer to 350 degrees F/180 degrees C.
7. Transfer the batter into a small air fryer baking pan. Then gently tap the pan on a table to release all of the air bubbles.
8. Cover the pan with some aluminum foil, tightly, and then poke some holes into the foil.
9. Reduce heat to 325 degrees F/160 degrees C, and bake for about 35 minutes. Then remove the foil and bake for another 5 minutes, until it is golden brown.
10. Let it cool completely before removing it from the pan.

Chapter 5: Fruit-Filled Goodness

Banana Bread

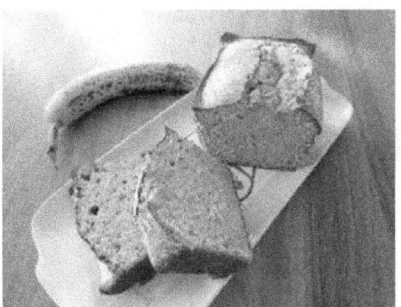

Yield: 4 to 6 servings

Time to make: about 1 1/2 hours

Ingredients:
- 1/4 cup of butter
- 2 tablespoons of honey
- 1 banana, mashed

- 1 cup of self-rising flour
- 1 egg
- 1/2 teaspoon of cinnamon
- 1/3 cup of brown sugar
- a pinch of salt, to taste
- nonstick cooking spray

Directions:

1. Preheat the air fryer to 325 degrees F/160 degrees C.
2. Spray air fryer baking pan with nonstick spray.
3. In a mixing bowl, beat the brown sugar and butter until creamy. Then add the honey, egg, banana, cinnamon, flour and salt, and mix thoroughly until smooth.
4. Transfer the batter to the pan and then use a spoon or spatula to even the top out.
5. Bake in the air fryer for 30 minutes, until a toothpick inserted into the center comes out clean.

Mini Pumpkin Pies

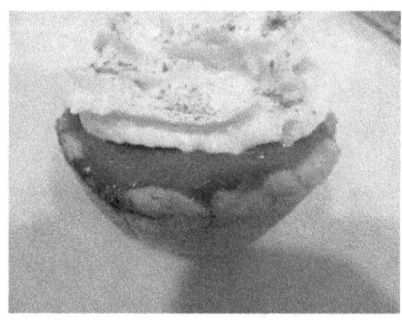

Yield: 9 servings

Time to make: 35 minutes

Ingredients:

For the Pumpkin Filling:

- 1 29-ounce can of pumpkin
- 4 eggs, slightly beaten
- 1 1/2 cups of sugar
- 1 teaspoon of salt
- 2 teaspoons of ground cinnamon

- 1 teaspoon of ginger
- 3/4 teaspoon of nutmeg
- 1/2 teaspoon of cloves
- 2 12-ounce cans of evaporated milk

For the Mini Crusts:

- 1/2 cup of flour
- 2 1/3 tablespoons of butter + additional for greasing the pastry cases
- 1/2 ounce of castor sugar
- water

Directions:

For the Pumpkin Filling:

(Note: you will probably have filling leftover, which can be used for anything else you want.)

1. Combine all of the pumpkin filling ingredients into a bowl and then mix thoroughly.

For the Mini Crusts:

2. Preheat the air fryer to 350 degrees F/180 degrees C.
3. In a mixing bowl using clean hands, rub the butter into the plain flour. Then mix the sugar well into it. Next, add enough water until the ingredients become a moist dough. Knead the dough until it has a texture that I smooth.
4. Grease the silicone pastry case(s) with butter, then spread out the dough into the pastry cases.
5. Fill each case to about 4/5 (about 80%) full with the pumpkin filling.
6. Bake in the air fryer for about 15 minutes.
7. Remove and let rest for five minutes or so before removing the pies to cool on a cooling rack.

Scrumptious Apple Pie

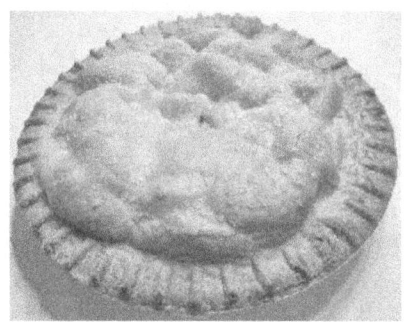

Yield: 6 servings

Time to make: 1 hour 20 minutes

Ingredients:

For the Pie Crust:

- 2 1/2 cups of all-purpose flour
- 1 cup of unsalted butter, chilled and then cut into tablespoon-size pieces
- 1/2 teaspoon of salt
- 7 tablespoons of ice water
- 1 tablespoon of cider vinegar

For the Apple Filling:

- cooking spray
- 1 large apple, chopped
- 2 teaspoons of lemon juice
- 1 tablespoon of ground cinnamon
- 2 tablespoons of sugar
- 1/2 teaspoon of vanilla extract
- 1 tablespoon of butter
- 1 egg, beaten
- 1 tablespoon of raw sugar

Directions:

First, prepare the pie crust as follows:

1. Using a food processor, combine the flour, salt and butter until the mixture turns into something like coarse crumbs.
2. In a separate small bowl, stir together the vinegar and water.

3. Pour half of the water-vinegar mix into the food processor and pulse to combine. Then add the remaining and pulse until the mixture just comes together.
4. Transfer this dough onto a work surface and then shape it into a round dough and divide it in half. Then make each half into a disc that's about five inches wide.
5. Wrap each disc with plastic wrap and then place in the fridge for at least 30 minutes before use.

After 30 minutes, prepare the pie and filling as follows:

6. Preheat the air fryer to the highest temperature possible.
7. Spray a air fryer baking container with cooking spray. Then press one of the crust dough discs into a small pie tin and then trim it off leaving an extra 1/8 of an inch hanging over.
8. Cut the second crust dough disc to a little smaller than the size of your baking basket. Set aside.
9. Place the apple, lemon juice, cinnamon, sugar and vanilla extract in a bowl and mix to combine. Then pour the apple mixture into your pie tin. Top with the pieces of butter.
10. Place the second piece of crust dough on top and pinch the edges shut. Then use a knife to make a few slits into the top of the pie.
11. Brush the beaten egg onto the top of the crust and then sprinkle the raw sugar over the egg.
12. Reduce heat to 320 degrees F/160 degrees C, carefully place the pie into the air fryer basket, and bake at this temperature for 30 minutes.

Fantasmic Fruit Jam Tarts

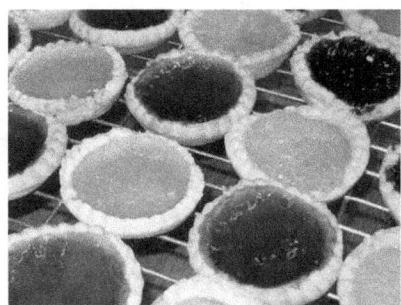

Yield: 9 servings

Time to make: 18 minutes

Ingredients:
- 1 1/2 cups of plain flour
- 1/2 cup of butter
- 1/8 cup of castor sugar
- jam of choice, such as strawberry, orange, etc.
- water

Directions:
1. Preheat the air fryer to 350 degrees F/180 degrees C.
2. In a bowl, rub the butter into the sugar and flour until you get coarse crumbs.
3. Then add water a little at a time until you have a pastry dough that is firm.
4. Grease 9 silicone pastry cases. Then divide the dough up and put them into the cases to make 9 tarts.
5. Place about 2 tablespoons of jam into each case.
6. Bake in the air fryer for about 10 minutes, until the pastry is cooked.

Cinnamon Apple Samosas

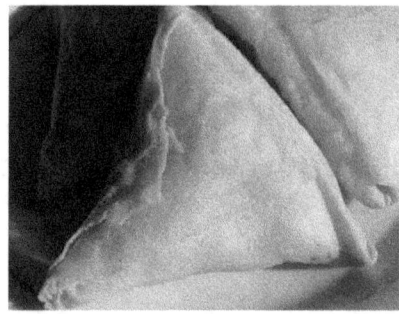

Yield: 5 servings

Time to make: 10 minutes

Ingredients:
- 3 apples, peeled and then chopped into small pieces
- 3 tablespoons of raisins
- 3 tablespoons of brown sugar
- 3 dashes of cinnamon
- 3 dashes of nutmeg

- 3 squirts of butter spray
- 10 fill pastry sheets
- 5 tablespoons of oil or additional butter spray

Directions:

1. Preheat the air fryer to 400 degrees F/200 degrees C.
2. In a large mixing bowl, mix together the apples, raisins, brown sugar, cinnamon and nutmeg, along with three squirts of the butter spray.
3. Fill each pastry sheet with some of the filling and then fold it up into triangles.
4. Brush a bit of oil onto both sides of each samosa, or spray each with some butter spray.
5. Fry in the air fryer until they are golden brown, about 5 minutes or less.

Lovely Lemon Bars

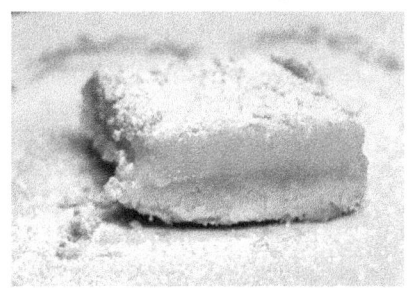

Yield: 9 servings

Time to make: about 45 minutes

Ingredients:

For the Base:

- 1/2 cup of flour
- 1/4 cup of sugar
- 2 ounces of butter

For the Filling:

- 2 eggs,
- 3/4 cup of sugar
- lemon juice from 1 to 2 lemons
- 1/4 cup of flour

- icing sugar, for dusting the tops of the bars

Directions:

For the Base:

1. Preheat the air fryer to 325 degrees F/160 degrees C.
2. Combine the flour and sugar in a bowl. Then add in the butter and use an electric mixer to mix well.
3. Press the resulting mixture into the bottom of an air fryer baking pan and bake for 15 minutes. Remove temporarily but keep the temperature at 325 degrees F/160 degrees F.

For the Filling:

4. In a bowl, whisk the eggs and sugar until smooth. Then stir in the lemon juice. Next, add the flour and mix well.
5. Pour this filling on top of the base, and then place back in the air fryer to bake for another 20 minutes.
6. Remove and cool for about 30 minutes before dusting the top of the filling with icing sugar and then cutting it into squares.

Raisin Bread Pudding

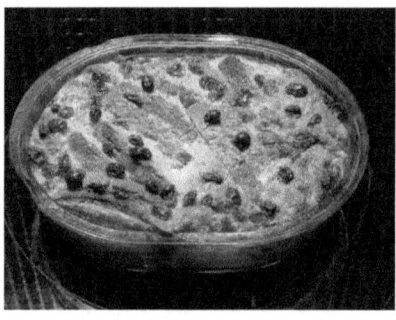

Yield: 2 servings

Time to make: 35 to 40 minutes

Ingredients:

- 2 slices of bread of choice
- 2 tablespoons of raisins, soaked in hot water for 15 minutes
- 1 cup of milk
- 1 egg
- 1 tablespoon of brown sugar
- 1/2 teaspoon of ground cinnamon

- 1/4 teaspoon of vanilla essence

Directions:

1. In a bowl, beat the egg. Then add the milk, vanilla, ground cinnamon and sugar, and mix well. Finally, add the raisins.
2. Cut the bread into 14 cubes each slice, and then place it in an air fryer baking basket.
3. Pour the egg mixture over it and place in the fridge to soak for 15 to 20 minutes.
4. Once done soaking, add a little more sugar to the top.
5. Preheat the air fryer 350 degrees F/180 degrees C for 3 minutes.
6. Bake the pudding for 12 minutes, checking after 10 to make sure it's not too brown in color. Adjust temperature and/or time as necessary according to preference in doneness.

Conclusion

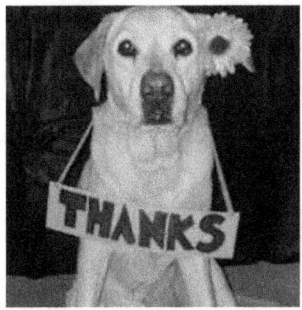

Thank you again for downloading this book! I hope you learned a lot and have found great, new ways to use your air fryer!

Thank you and good luck!

Part 2

Introduction

Amidst the constant boom of technology, new things are always coming to our home that promise to simplify or improve our lives. Now, it is the turn of the air fryer. There is widespread debate about whether this device really is improving our health, or simply an overly marketed gimmick.

The main premise of an air fryer is that we do not need to immerse our food for an extended period in large amounts of oil to obtain that incredible flavor and crunchy texture we crave. With only half a tablespoon of oil and 10 or 15 minutes we can achieve the same delicious results.

Though most of the foods prepared with this cooking device do not require oil at all, only hot air. Based on "Rapid Air" technology, air fryers blow superheated air around to cook foods that would traditionally be fried in oil.

To begin to understand this controversial debate, we must first understand how different types of air fryers work, and how to use them. .

What Are The Benefits Of An Air Fryer?

French fries are part of the Belgian tradition, and nowhere is it written that this golden delight should be cooked in astronomical quantities of oil. And why is it necessary that your kitchen still smell like them the next day? It's no wonder the air fryer is so successful.

1. Faster and more economical

The combination of the heating element and the circulation of hot air allows your food to cook faster in an air fryer than in a traditional oven. That's why this device should not only be seen as a healthier alternative to a fryer, but also as a more economical alternative to baking.

2. Preheating becomes obselete

Unlike deep fryers and most ovens, preheating is not necessary with an air fryer. This saves time and allows you to prepare snacks more spontaneously. Though in the case of some models, preheating for a few minutes can reduce cooking time even further.

3. Neither shake nor return

Hot air, possibly accompanied by a stroke of oil, passes through the food at high speed and cooks all sides of the food evenly. You will not have to shake or return your food.

4. Safer

An air fryer not only eliminates the risk of hot oil or grease splashing, but it's a closed cooking environment. This well-insulated design minimizes the risk of burns and other accidents. An air fryer is ideal if you are not comfortable using a traditional fryer.

5. More ecological

The air that is rejected by the device goes through a series of filters. They ensure that this air contains no harmful substances or unpleasant odors. It's good for the environment, and your cooking.

6. You choose the oil

You use the oil of your choice, according to your taste or recipe. This can be olive oil, peanut, sunflower, or even butter spray.

7. Simultaneous cooking

The basket, which can be equipped with a separator often supplied with the appliance or sold separately, allows you to cook two preparations at the same time.

8. Welcome foil

You can use parchment paper, foil wraps or aluminum foil, but always make sure there is enough space for air to circulate evenly.

9. Easy cleaning

As there is less fat, and it all is collected in the preparation basket, cleaning becomes a breeze. This basket (and possibly the accessories) can go in the dishwasher. Many models also have an automatic cleaning function for the rest of the device.

10. No more calories

We have already emphasized this aspect, but we cannot mention the benefits of the air fryer without mentioning the fact that foods - especially, but not only, fried - absorb less fat, are less caloric and are therefore better for your health.

OTHER BENEFITS

Calorie reduction: one of the main benefits attributed to these appliances is the considerable decrease in fat consumption. Unquestionably when frying food in deep oil we add many calories, so one of the most attractive benefits of an air fryer is the elimination of these extra calories. In proportion, we use only 80-85% of the oil that we would use with the equivalent conventional frying method.

Reduction in cooking time: With the programming of temperature and time, we can control the constant flow of hot air and accelerate the process of cooking food. It delivers time savings of up to 40% compared to a regular frying process.

Reduction of energy expenditure: If we compare the energy consumption of the air fryer with that of a standard electric oven, we can see that the consumption of energy is much lower. You reduce energy cost by more than 50% when using the air fryer. For example, the Philips Air Fryer consumes about 390Wh to fry half a kilo of potatoes - that's 45% less electricity than a conventional oven uses! .

Saving money: By not using nearly as much oil, you will save a considerable amount of money.

Ease of cleaning: With an air fryer, the cleaning process is much faster, or even non existent, depending on whether you want to spray oil (to flavor it) or not, on the food to be cooked. The container where the food is placed is removable, which makes it easy to wash and clean.

Based on all this, we can conclude that having an air fryer brings many advantages and benefits, not only to your health. Space inside the kitchen and time savings are other considerable benefits to be had, combined with the fact that air fryers are not limited to just frying food, as we can control both temperature and timing. This allows us to steam and cook as well, both of these also being significant benefits of having this appliance. Especially if we do not have fried foods in our regular diet. These two cooking methods can also be achieved in less time than with other, traditional kitchen implements.

Having such a versatile kitchen implement allows us to be more creative and vary our diet more frequently. This empowers us to have a more regularly balanced diet, without so much effort. The air fryer allows us to cook steamed vegetables, make roasted chicken, french fries, and countless other recipes - only limited by your creativity!

Is It As Healthy As You Think?

Most of my patients love using their air fryers. These countertop devices circulate heat at high temperatures to fry, grill, or bake without using oil. They create a crispy outside layer while leaving food moist and chewy on the inside.

The good news is that, overall, air-frying has more benefits than drawbacks.

The upside

The main reason people love air-frying is that, compared with deep-frying, it significantly reduces overall calorie intake. Most people reduce their calorie intake by 70 to 80 percent, on average, when using air fryers.

Air fryers are also time-efficient. You can bake a chicken breast faster in an air fryer than you can in your oven, and clean-up is typically easier.

Another benefit: If you have picky vegetable eaters at home (I'm thinking of kids, in particular), air-frying is a great way to crisp up veggies and make them tastier.

Lastly, unlike deep-frying, air-frying typically won't fill your home with the smell of fried foods for hours.

The downside

One drawback to air-frying is that it prompts some people to think, "This is great — I can eat fried food every day!"

Although a low-fat, air-fried diet sounds enticing, you'd end up missing out on the wonderful benefits of plant-based fats such as avocado oil and olive oil. (It's easy to forget that high-quality fat, in moderation, is critical for brain and hormone health.)

Air-frying also produces high temperatures at a very rapid rate, thus making it extremely easy to burn food, and charred food may be carcinogenic.

Also, because most devices only cook 1 to 3 pounds of food at a time, it can be challenging to air-fry meals for a large family.

The best foods to air-fry

Any foods you're used to frying, like potatoes and chicken, generally turn out well in the air fryer.

If you're looking for something to air-fry, I'd recommend home-made sweet potato fries. It can be challenging to make them crispy in a conventional oven. Instead, sprinkle them with your favorite seasoning, throw them in the air fryer, and enjoy!

One last thought: If you want to invest in an air fryer, I'd recommend looking for models that use BPA-free plastic.

Fryer Without Oil Which One To Buy?

If you are evaluating the purchase of an oil-free fryer or air fryer, you'll want to do a comparison. To prepare this review, we have used customer opinions, sales rankings, and our own experience. If you have already used any of the models reviewed or wish to share your experience with another brand, we would be delighted to hear from you.

Yes, an oil-free fryer will be consistent with your purpose of preparing healthy cooking, with fewer calories. Every day we are busier cooking healthy meals, choosing the best ingredients, and balancing our diets to include all kinds of foods.

You love healthy food, you cook steamed foods regularly, but you miss fried foods, especially their flavor. Well, there is a solution, a product that will allow you to cook with hardly any oil (reducing its use by 80%) or without any oil: oil-free deep fryers or hot air fryer.

We say to cook and not to fry since, speaking with propriety, the fryer without oil does not brown.

It works similarly to an oven, but in a much more practical and fast way and of course, with lower energy consumption.

How does an oil-free fryer or hot air fryer work?

Its operating principle is similar to an oven, and it cooks through the circulation of fast moving hot air. An oil-free fryer is formed by the container, (which is the one that determines the capacity and where you need to evaluate what volume you need) time, and temperature controls.

What foods can you prepare in a fryer without oil?

Undoubtedly one of the first dishes you can imagine is french fries, but you can also prepare fish, nuggets, empanadillas, chicken, skewers, etc. Even fried eggs!

Remember that the principle of these devices makes them a deep fryer with little oil, maintaining the flavor, but without adding calories.

Other options for cooking without oil, have you thought about them?

Have you ever wondered what other cooking utensils can help you cook without oil? As an example, a good nonstick skillet allows you to cook without oil, getting effects similar to those mentioned to those with a fryer without oil.

To choose the best fryer without oil, keep these tips in mind

Yes, it is good to analyze several points when deciding on the best oil-free fryer for your home, not just the price, capacity, or energy consumption.

Seven aspects to analyze in your choice:

Price: the price is the number 1 criterion but not the only one you should consider. Think of it like an investment, perhaps go a little higher than you initially intended on and enjoy good results in the long term.

Warranty: Who responds if you have any problems? Having official technical service support is always a plus.

Capacity: for how many people do you usually cook? Think about this point to not buy something too big or too small for your day to day needs.

Dimensions: (necessary space in the kitchen) where are you going to store the air fryer? We know that there is not always space in the kitchen ... think about where you are going to keep it.

Spare Parts: Do you intend to use it until it breaks and then throw it away? Don't! Choose appliances that can be repaired to extend their life.

Consumption: the power it uses will appear on your electricity bill ... keep that in mind.

Previous user opinions: a must in any current purchase is to know the experience of prior users, and their evaluation of its actual use.

The five best air fryers

To present these five options, we have evaluated the experience, price, and quantities of commonly sold models sold in Spain.

Russell Hobbs air fryer

In this case, we have selected the Purifry Russell Hobbs model. Located in the mid-range of prices, it has a high demand in Spain. It is a powerful machine and is well-liked by its users.

The Russell Hobbs brand has official representation in Spain and has an authorized technical service support team:

- Dimensions: Width 32.8 cm, Length 32 cm. High 38.4 cm
- Price: 140 euro, approximately
- Quality approved by Test Magazine

Philips air fryer

Our top choice. The Phillips brand is trendy, accessible, and has points of sale and technical service throughout the world. The Philips Airfryer is the most popular in Europe, and the one we consider to have the best price/quality ratio:

- Dimensions: Width 28.7 cm, Length 38 cm. 32 cm high
- Available accessories
- Price: 180 euros, approximately

Lidl air fryer

The Silvercrest fryer marketed by LIDL has good reviews and is available at the lowest price point. Its quality of materials and performance is good, although it is below the other models. It is a good choice for occasional use:

- Dimensions: Width 28.7 cm, Length 38 cm. 32 cm high
- Price: 70 euros, approximately
- Where you can buy it: only in LIDL stores and for limited periods of time.

Actifry Tefal air fryer

The Tefal Actifry fryer is the most complete, large, and powerful option. The Tefal brand is recognized worldwide and has points of sale and technical service:

- Dimensions: Width 48 cm, Length 38.6 cm. High 31 cm.
- Available accessories
- Price: 200 euros, approximately

Princess oil-free fryer

The Princess Aerofryer XL model is the one with the greatest capacity compared here. It is a lower price than most of its competitors and you can buy it online. Princess is a brand of Princess Household Appliances BV, of the Netherlands:

- Dimensions: Width 38 cm, Length 34 cm. 34 cm high
- Digital remote
- Price: 110 euros, approximately

Your experience with an air fryer

In addition to what we propose we would like to read your experiences with the use of your appliance, is it worth buying? What experience have you had with the Russell Hobbs, Lidl, Phillips, Tefal, or Princess models?

Many people doubt whether it is worth buying an air fryer if you can do the same type of cooking without one. The reality is that it depends on each home and the kind of cuisine you choose. In Europe, fried foods are the order of the day, many dishes go through oil, and having an alternative that reduces calories is good news.

Another point to consider before buying is the space they will occupy. We have included this data in the comparison so you can get an idea of their dimensions and understand whether you can incorporate them into your kitchen.

What Should You Keep In Mind Before Buying An Air Fryer

1. Type of frying basket

Baskets that can be removed entirely to be washed more easily are generally preferable, as in the models I chose for this comparison. The material is also essential: while the metallic ones distribute the heat more quickly, the ceramic ones are easier to clean. Some models combine the best of both worlds and offer the option of metal baskets with non-stick coatings.

2. Capacity

This will depend on the amount of food you can prepare in a single cycle of your fryer. It is generally not necessary to have one of a large size, but if your family is enormous, or you usually cook for several days at a time, it is better that you choose one of the models with a higher capacity, some of which can even roast a whole chicken!

3. Preset programs

Many offer presets for some of the most common foods such as chips, roast chicken, pie, steak, roasts, and more. They are very convenient since, with the press of a button, you will get food cooked to perfection. Some models even allow you to make custom programs and store them in their memory.

4. Programmable timer / start

Since we are modernizing the kitchen, it is worth choosing a model that allows you to schedule the exact time at which the food begins to be prepared, so that it is freshly made at precisely the time you sit at the table. On many occasions, I leave everything prepared inside the fryer and go out to do my homework, with the assurance that it will start cooking at the right time so that lunch is ready when I return.

5. Preheating time

Some old fryers needed up to 10 minutes to start cooking your food adequately, making you waste time and consuming more energy than necessary. Fortunately, this is no longer the case with newer models and I have been careful to choose products that begin to heat almost immediately for this comparison.

Air Fryer Vs. Oven

Should you spend money on a dean air fryer, or does the "frying" of the oven produce the same level of crispiness? We will investigate.

The fryer is right on the heels of the Instant Pot skirts in terms of popularity among home cooks, as an appliance that can "do it all." So what exactly is an air fryer? It is essentially a compact convection oven that cooks food at very high temperatures while dry air circulates with a built-in fan. Its key selling point is that it drastically reduces the amount of oil used during the frying to achieve crispy results. Since these devices can be quite expensive, I decided to try one and see what all the fuss was about. I tried two variations of "fried chicken": breaded and without bread. Both chicken variations were cooked in the dean sr42g air fryer and a conventional convection oven. I wanted to know if it was worth the high price, or if I should just stick to the oven.

There are a handful of different fryers on the market that range from $ 70 to $200. I used the Gourmia GTA2500 model for the test. When I opened the box, the amount of parts and accessories involved was a bit overwhelming. It took me a while to analyze everything and find out what parts I needed and which were superfluous. Once assembled, the fryer looked like a mini spaceship! Quite bulky and dome-like, I'm not quite sure how I would feel if I had this on the kitchen counter, but I'm getting side tracked here. I ended up using only the cooking rack and the frying basket for the fryer.

While preparing the chicken without bread, I prepared the oven to preheat to 400 ° F, which already highlights a benefit of the dhg fryer: it does not require preheating. Typically, to "fry" in the oven, you want the oven to be at a very high temperature, thus heating your kitchen. The fryer saves you from an unbearably hot kitchen; however, it emits a much louder noise than any oven when it is in operation.

When I started loading the chicken in the fryer basket, I realized that I was only going to be able to place four pieces in it, maybe five if I pressed it in.

Then, I needed to cook two batches for the same amount of chicken in the oil-free fryer that I could cook in a single batch in the oven. Since the fryer only can prepare food in small quantities, it is probably more suitable for those who cook for 1-2 people. If you are cooking for more people, you may want to skip the fryer and go straight to the oven.

Once the chicken was in the frying basket, I press the "fry" button that adjusts the fryer to a temperature of 390 ° F for 30 minutes. I found the configuration accurate, so I didn't fix it. I started with the breadless chicken, and let it run the full 30 minutes. For the oven, I lined a frying pan with aluminum foil and placed it on a rack on the sheet. I baked the chicken on the rack and put it in the oven at the same time I prepared the fryer. The fryer works with a timer and turns off when the food is ready, decreasing the possibility of burning the food or cooking too much. When the air stops circulating in the air fryer, the cooking process stops, unlike a hot oven that has recently been turned off and remains hot.

I was delighted with the results of the fryer. The chicken was beautifully golden, with crispy edges, but still very moist inside. And I was ready for the table before the oven batch (which took around 35 to 40 minutes). When I took the chicken out of the oven, it was a little less crispy, but it was still quite moist inside. I tossed the two batches in a sweet peach barbecue sauce to finish. For me, the benefit of the double gas fryer in this round of "frying" was that it technically cooked the chicken faster. The downside was that I could only use half the amount of chicken compared to the oven.

The breaded chicken that I "fried" was a little more interesting.

I followed Leah Chasereceta's baked, fried chicken recipe for the second batch of chicken. After dredging, I brushed each piece of chicken with a light layer of olive oil to absorb the flour and prevent it from cracking and not "frying" properly. I adjusted the fryer to 410 ° F for 30 minutes and preheated the oven to 425 ° F. However, after 10 minutes of cooking, the oven started smoking very severely, so I reduced the temperature to 400 ° F. (I suspect that the excess flour in the pan was burning). Halfway through cooking, I dumped the chicken in the oven and the fryer and noticed that the bottom breading was glued to the basket in the aeg double fryer, so I would recommend spraying the bucket with cooking spray. Naturally, It took the oven batch 15 minutes longer (45 minutes in total) to cook since I lowered the temperature.

The chicken fryer again cooked faster, was more relaxed, and did not smoke in the kitchen. The batch from the air fryer was deliciously crispy, and the empanada was cooked entirely, with no raw pieces to be seen. The drawback, again, was that it could only cook a few pieces of chicken at a time.

That said, although the outside of the empanada may not have been very crispy, the meat was very juicy.

Just for fun, I also tried a bag of frozen fries. I should have paid a little more attention because they ended up a little too golden, but they were crispy. If perhaps a bit too crunchy...

Overall, I think this air fryer does an excellent job of cooking in small batches, and I enjoyed experimenting with it. Though admittedly, this appliance would be better for a home of one or two people. It would also be ideal to use as a portable oven when traveling. The main benefits of the double carrefour air fryer are:

- It allows you to significantly reduce the amount of oil that you would typically use during frying.
- You can open and close it during the cooking process without risk of burning.
- It cooks faster than a traditional oven.
- Cleaning was super easy and painless.

If you are interested in trying an anionic fryer, the Philips AirFryer seems to be a popular model on Amazon. You can also check the Gourmia GTA2500 model for $ 179.99 that I used during the tests.

Air Fryer Recipes

1. Fish in Air Fryer

Ingredients

- 1 lemon's juice
- 3 fish fillets
- 1 tbsp full seasoning with achiote
- 1 tbsp ground garlic
- 1 tbsp ground onion
- Chickpea flour
- Water

Preparation

20 minutes

Rinse the fish. And cut into pieces. Dry with paper towels. Spread lemon juice and seasoning.

In a bowl, add the chickpea flour and a little water to form a thick cream.

Batter the fish pieces. Spread the pan of the fryer with oil and place the fish in it. Cook according to the instructions listed on your specific fryer.

The cooking time will depend on the equipment you use.

2. Wings in air fryer

Ingredients

- 1 Kg wings, split into 2 batches
- 50 g flour
- 1 tsp paprika powder
- 1 tsp olive oil
- Salt and pepper to taste

Preparation

Clean and dry the wings with water.
Coat in flour
Spread the oil over the wings
Sprinkle paprika with pepper and salt to taste
Place in the fryer for 15min at 360º F

3. Gluten-free yogurt cake in air fryer

You can make delicious sponge cake without gluten in an air fryer.

Ingredients

- Greek yogurt
- 3 eggs
- 150 g sugar
- 100 g cream
- 50 g sunflower oil
- 50 g butter
- 200 g gluten free flour
- Salt
- yeast

Preparation

Put the eggs, yogurt and sugar in the Thermomix. Mix well. Add the rest of the ingredients and mix again.

Put the dough in the sponge cake container, previously brushed with oil. Preheat the fryer and put the mold with the dough in it for 40 minutes at 170º.

When it cools, remove from mold and decorate to taste.

4 Mini Tatin cake in the air fryer

Ingredients

- 100 g flour
- 50 g cold butter
- 25 ml water
- 1 pinch salt
- 1 apple
- Lemon juice
- 25 g sugar
- 15 g butter

Preparation

40 minutes

1. The first thing to do is prepare the dough. For this we put the salt in the flour, and add the cold butter. Then mix everything until it looks like sand.
2. Now add 25 ml of water and mix until it is a homogeneous mass that does not stick to your hands. Wrap it in a transparent paper and set aside.
3. In a clay pot we mix the sugar and butter and let it melt.
4. Now core and peel the apple, then apply the lemon juice so that it does not go brown, you can alternatively leave it in water with lemon.
5. When our sugar and butter are golden, we put the apples on top, placing them tightly, to cover the entire surface.
6. Leave the caramelized apples for 15 to 20 minutes, we will come back to them.
7. Meanwhile, we stretch the dough, using a rolling pin and baking paper.
8. Once the apples are caramelized, we cover them with the broken dough. Cut off whatever is left over. We also puncture the center with a fork to give the steam a hole to vent through.
9. Preheat the fryer to 160 degrees, and put the cake in for about 15 minutes.
10. After this, let it set at room temperature for a while to enable you to remove it easily. Run a knife around the edges and turn it to loosen. Enjoy !

5 Rabas in hot air fryer

Ingredients

- 16 rabas

- 1 egg
- Bread crumbs
- Condiments: salt, pepper, sweet paprika

Preparation

In my case they were frozen so I put them in hot water and then boiled for 2 minutes.

Remove and dry well.

Beat the egg and season to taste. I put salt, pepper and sweet paprika on mine. Place in the egg.

Spray with fritolin and cook for 5 more minutes at 200 degrees.

6. Spanish potatoes in hot air fryer

Ingredients

- 400 g potato
- Water
- 1 tablespoon olive oil
- Salt

Preparation

1. Peel and cut the potato into julienne pieces, about 0.5 CM thick.
2. Prepare a bowl with very cold water, if necessary add ice. Place the cut potatoes in it for at least 30 minutes to make them starchy.
3. Dry each potato with an absorbent napkin and place in another dry bowl.
4. When they are all dry, sprinkle with oil or brush with olive oil and season with salt and whatever you like (sweet paprika, oregano, etc).
5. Place in air fryer without oil at 160 degrees for 17 minutes. Then stir
6. Set the fryer to 180 degrees for another 10 minutes, and that's it!
7. To make in an electric oven place a butter paper and on it and separate the potatoes from each other. Cook at the same temperature for the same time. Remove from the oven after 17 minutes, remove the paper, turn and cook for another 10 minutes at 180 degrees.
8. If you dare to do them I would love to hear your experience!

7. Breaded prawns in hot air fryer

Ingredients

- 9 raw prawns

- 1 egg
- Bread crumbs
- Condiments: salt, pepper and sweet paprika

Preparation

1. As the prawns were clean, but raw and frozen I simply put mine in water and let them boil for 2 minutes.
2. Remove from water and dry with absorbent paper.
3. Beat the egg and season to taste. In my case as my daughter would be sharing this, I did not add anything spicy. Place them on a stick of brochettes and brush with beaten egg. Leave in the egg until breading.
4. Coat with breadcrumbs. Brush again with egg and repeat this process.
5. Place in the fryer strainer. Cook for 5 minutes at 160 degrees. Remove.
6. Spray with fritolin or brush with oil. Place for 5 more minutes in the fryer at 200 degrees. Enjoy!

8. Pizzetas in fryer without oil

Ingredients

- 250 g flour
- g salt
- 1 pinch sugar
- 1/2 packet of instant yeast
- 150ml warm water
- 1 dash of olive oil
- sauce
- 1/2 onion
- Ketchup
- Ham
- Mozzarella

Preparation

1. Put the flour in a bowl with the salt salt and a drizzle of olive oil, add the warm water and knead.
2. Leave in the bowl in a warm place to rise

3. Then divide the dough into 4 and knead on discs that enter the fryer pan without oil. Cut shortening paper on discs.
4. Place the dough on the paper and add the ham and cheese sauce.
5. Put in a pan for about 7 minutes.

9   Wings with fine herbs without oil (in the fryer without oil)

Ingredients

3 people
- 1 kilo wings
- 1 envelope of thin herb magui
- The juice of a lemon
- Salt

Preparation

40 minutes
1. Marinate the wings with the spices and the lemon, leave for 1 hour.
2. Set the fryer to preheat for about 10 minutes, at 200 degrees.
3. Put the wings in the bucket and stir occasionally, take out and serve.
4. An easy and healthy recipe without any oil!

10 Bondiola chopped (air fryer)

Ingredients

- 1 kg bondiola in pieces
- Bread crumbs
- 2 eggs
- Seasoning to taste

Preparation

1. Cut the bondiola into small pieces, seasoning to taste.
2. Beat the eggs.
3. Add beaten egg and then breadcrumbs to bondiola.
4. Place in the air fryer for 20 minutes, turning half way through.

11. Zucchini sticks in oil-free fryer / oven

Ingredients

- 16 apx canes
- 1 zucchini
- 2 eggs
- flour
- 1 lemon
- grated cheese and breadcrumbs

Preparation

1. Cut off the tips of the zucchini and chop into sticks (or slices if desired).
2. Fill a bowl with flour, another with peppered eggs, and one more with lemon zest, grated cheese, and breadcrumbs mixed together.
3. Coat the zucchini in flour, then egg, and finally with the mixture of lemon, cheese and breadcrumbs.
4. Add to fryer without oil, or preheated oven, for approx. 20 min. Serve warm and with soy sauce or ketchup.

12. Pumpkin croquettes using oil-free fryer

Ingredients

- Pumpkin puree
- 1 onion
- 1 tbsp or 2 tbsp grated cheese
- Eggs
- Bread crumbs
- Port health light cheese

Preparation

1. Make pumpkin puree.
2. Saute chopped onion.
3. Mix in a bowl the pumpkin, grated cheese, onion, salt, pepper, and nutmeg.
4. Assemble the croquettes, and cover with cheese (I use port health light), then coat with beaten egg and breadcrumbs.

5. Coat air fryer with vegetable oil spray, and cook at 200 degrees for 20 minutes.

13. 4D turbocecofry iron knives, dietary fryer

Ingredients

- 1 set of living knives
- The juice of a lime
- Very finely chopped fresh parsley
- 4 cloves garlic, minced
- Salt maldom on scales
- Fat salt to clean the razors

Preparation

1. We soak the razors with fat salt to release the sand. It is best to put them vertically (I have not done so) for a minimum of 20 minutes
2. Mix the ingredients for the dressing
3. We rinse and drain the knives. We coat the bucket with the dressing with the help of a silicone brush. We coat the knives and leave them until they have a beautiful golden color. In three minutes they are ready but I like to leave them a little longer until golden (about 8 minutes). Paint with the dressing a couple of times, at least, during the process.
4. Serve with maldom salt, broken between fingers

These are delicious and when made in the turbocecofry do not stain anything and do not leave a lingering smell..

14. Spiced chicken wings, in oil-free fryer

Ingredients

4 portions

- 1 Kg chicken wings
- Salt
- 1 teaspoon paprika
- Garlic powder
- Freshly ground pepper
- 1/2 teaspoon curry
- 1/2 teaspoon turmeric

Preparation

50 minutes

1. Clean and defeather the wings well, if they had them, discard the tips and cut them in two, add the salt, and make a mixture with the rest of the spices, smear the wings well, then let them marinate a little.
2. Plug in the Cecofry oil-free fryer, or whichever one you use. Add the wings and leave them for 45 minutes in the fryer, the result is very crispy and very tasty wings.

I hope you like them, they are great!

15. Grilled squid with jocca oil-free fryer

Ingredients

1 serving
- medium squids
- 2 tbsp extra virgin olive oil
- 1 clove garlic
- parsley

Preparation

15 minutes
1. Clean the squid and season.
2. Coat well with 1 tsp of oil, using your to ensure it is well coated on all sides.
3. Place them inside the fryer basket and program 200º, cook for 10 minutes.
4. In a bowl, we combine the other oil with minced garlic and a little parsley, stir everything well.
5. Toss the oil with the garlic and eat!

I accompanied them with steamed potatoes and salad, to create a rich and healthy meal!

16. French fries and Iberian pork fillets in a fryer without jocca oil

Ingredients

2 portions
- big potatoes
- 4 Iberian prey fillets
- 1 tbsp olive oil
- 1 pinch sweet paprika
- Salt

Preparation

35 minutes

1. Peel the potatoes, wash and cut for frying.
2. Put in the basket of the fryer with half a tablespoon of oil, salt and paprika, program 200º and cook for 15 minutes, stirring halfway through.
3. When finished, remove and keep warm.
4. We put the seasoned fillets in the basket and brush with the rest of the oil, then cook at 200º for 10 minutes.
5. This will create a super light, healthy and delicious dinner with the potatoes.

17. Roasted apples in Jocca oil-free fryer

Ingredients

4 portions

- 4 apples
- 4 ctas dulce de leche
- ice cream to serve, and mint to garnish

Preparation

20 minutes

1. Wash the apples and take out a large part of the applesauce.
2. Add a whole can of dulce de leche (you can also use sugar and a little muscatel).
3. Put them in the basket and program 180º, cooking for 18 minutes. When the time ends, see if they are ready. You may have to cook for 2 more minutes.
4. Let cool and serve with lemon ice cream and mint leaves. A healthy, quick and delicious rich dessert.

18. Chard fritters with Electric Fryer

Ingredients

4 portions

- 100 gr whole wheat flour
- 3 eggs
- 1 chard bouquet
- tablespoons mix seeds
- 1 tablespoon baking powder
- Salt

- Pepper
- 2 tablespoons olive oil
- 1 cup milk

Preparation

Wash the chard.

Cook the chard for a minute, then proceed to cut it thinly.

In a bowl place the three eggs with the milk and the seed and beat together.

Place the cut chard in the bowl, then add the flour, baking powder and oil.

Turn on the fryer, at about 180 °, you may need to wait a few minutes for it to warm up.

With the fritolin, brush the basket and place the previously prepared mixture inside with a spoon.

After a few minutes, turn the mix to brown on the other side.

19. Chicken fajitas

Ingredients

15 fajitas

- 15 tortillas for fajitas
- 1 packet of spices for fajitas
- 2 large onions
- 2 large peppers of different colors
- 4 large chicken breasts
- 1 tablespoon sweet paprika
- Stir Fry Oil
- Ketchup
- Salt
- 1 kilo chips
- Mayonnaise
- Oil

Preparation

1. Cut the chicken into thin strips.
2. In a deep skillet, heat a small amount of oil and, when it is very hot, brown the chopped chicken with a little salt.
3. Once it is golden, remove it from the heat and put it in a strainer to drain.

4. Fry the potatoes.
5. Cut the onions and peppers into strips.
6. In the same pan heat a splash of oil and when it is hot, fry the vegetables with a little salt.
7. When the vegetables are tender, incorporate the chicken, paprika, the spice for fajitas, and a squirt of ketchup.
8. Mix everything very well and cook a few more minutes.
9. To assemble the fajitas, take a tortilla, add some mayonnaise, the other toppings for the fajitas, some chips and optional, a little more ketchup, close the fajita and enjoy!

20. Fried cheese

Ingredients

- Light blue cheese
- Light cheese
- 2 eggs
- Flour
- Bread crumbs
- Frying oil
- Strawberry jam or red berries to accompany

Preparation

1. Prepare the eggs in a bowl, and the flour and breadcrumbs in two separate dishes.
2. Peel the cheeses, taking care not to break them and pass them through the flour to coat.
3. Beat the egg and pass the cheese through it, ensuring it is well covered.
4. Then we pass everything through the breadcrumbs and let stand for a few minutes.
5. Heat the fryer.
6. Brown the cheese and drain on absorbent paper. We accompany the cheeses with jam, preferably of red fruits or similar.
7. Enjoy this rich entree in good company, bon appetit!

21. Chicken fingers

Ingredients

- 1 chicken breast
- 1 glass milk
- pepper
- parsley
- minced garlic
- 2-3 eggs
- flour
- bread crumbs
- frying oil
- barbecue sauce to accompany

Preparation

1. The first thing we have to do is clean and chop the breast into strips.
2. We put the chicken in a bowl.
3. Cover with a glass of milk and leave for 45 minutes.
4. Put the eggs on a plate.
5. Add the parsley and ground garlic. Mix.
6. Drain the chicken.
7. Season the chicken strips.
8. Pass each strip through the flour.
9. Then pass through the beaten egg.
10. Pass through the breadcrumbs.
11. Let them rest for about 15 minutes.
12. Heat the fryer, you may need to fry them in several batches.
13. Once fried we transfer them to a plate with absorbent paper.

Serve and eat with your fingers, accompanied by barbecue sauce. Enjoy them in good company, bon appetit!

22. Cod fillet, and cocorita purslane sauce

Ingredients

2 portions

- 500 g cod fillets without bones or skin
- 2 gobelins
- 4 cloves garlic

- 1 plate of breadcrumbs
- a little salt, pepper, and dried basil
- 1/2 cauliflower
- 200 g spinach
- 1 L milk
- 1/2 dl oil
- 1 dl flour

Preparation

30 minutes

1. Peel the garlic cloves, press them, salt and add the peeled eggs, and a little pentacolor pepper, plus a spoonful of basil. Beat well and add to the fillets that you salted and peppered .... now bread them and let them dry a little.
2. Put the oil in the bottom of the pan, add the flour and a tablespoon of coarse salt, stir, and add the milk. Light the stove and set to low heat and turn on the fryer. Stir every minute or so, and while this is cooking cut the spinach and cauliflower, then add them. When it starts to boil, turn off the heat and fry them one by one.
3. After two minutes at 170 degrees they should be ready.

23. Stew Italian zucchini with golden potatoes

Ingredients

5 servings

- 2 large Italian zucchini
- 1 scallion
- 200 grams ground post
- 2 Moroccan bread
- grated cheese
- 4 sheets Gauda Cheese
- 1 glass or 1/2 glass Wine or beer
- 1/2 cup milk
- 2 eggs
- Garlic
- oil
- salt

- oregano
- dressing
- broth
- paprika
- medium potatoes cooked and cut into small pieces

Preparation

time 45 min

Cook the zucchini with plenty of water and salt for 20 minutes, or until tender.

Fry the scallion in the pan, along with 2 heads of garlic and paprika. Then add the meat and continue to fry. Add salt, gourmet broth, complete dressing, and oregano then cook with half a glass of white wine or beer.

Meanwhile take the Moroccan bread and soak it completely in 1 cup of milk or half a cup of milk then grate, then add the two eggs and mix.

Stew Italian zucchini with golden potatoes

Drain all the cooking water from the zucchini, you can pass them through the vegetable centrifuge. Grind with Minipimer and return to the pot over low heat and add the milk shake milk and bread mix, now add the meat and finally add Grated cheese and Gauda cheese in slices to taste, then mix and simmer for a few minutes.

Once the potatoes are cooked, remove them from the water and fry until golden brown

Now serve in a deep dish and enjoy.

24. Chicken Wings and Ham, with Chimichurri

Ingredients

2 portions

- Fryer or saucepan with enough oil. 190 °>
- 1 super tray
- Flour and 1 part Garbazo
- Salt pepper
- Super chimichurri sauce

Preparation

30 minutes

1. Turn on the fryer, sprinkle the ham and pass it through the flour mixed with chickpea flour. Fry this mixture, then allow to cool and place on absorbent paper.

2. Using a hot plate, heat the chimichurri and add to taste. (you can buy this from the supermarket, and it will last longer without spoiling)..

25. Goat cheese salad

Ingredients

1 serving
- 1 lettuce bud
- 1 package Super Smoked Salmon
- 1 anchovy in oil
- Salt
- 1 bottle of Balsamic oil from Modena
- 1 goat cheese curler
- 1 egg
- bread crumbs
- 1 deep fryer

Preparation

1. Cut the goat cheese into portions and pass it through the egg and breadcrumbs.
2. Cut the bud into 4 parts in width and put at the base of the plate with a pinch of salt, then add a little Smoked Salmon, then the Goat cheese, which we will have previously passed through the fryer at 190 °. Add half of 1 anchovy and some Balsamic Oil.
3. Garnish with nuts.

26. Pilar House Eggs

Ingredients

2 portions
- 2 medium onions, or to taste
- frying peppers
- 500 grams frying potatoes
- 4 eggs
- Salt
- Oil
- 1 fryer

Preparation

Cut the onions in julienne style and fry them a little, then fry the peppers and then cut the potatoes into slices.

Place everything in the fryer.

In a large pan, add a little oil, and everything we've fried before, add a little salt and beat the eggs, stir with a wooden spoon.

27. potato balls

Ingredients

5 portions (21 potato balls)

- large potatoes
- flour
- 2 beaten eggs
- bread crumbs
- salt and white pepper
- To saute the potato--
- Butter
- Asturian milk
- -Decoration of the dish -
- 2 sticks of celery
- flour
- Utensils that we are going to use--
- 2 pots, 1 sprig, 1 fork and a fryer.

Preparation

40 minutes

1. Put a pot of water on the stove with a little salt., Peel potatoes and, when the water is boiling, add them. Cook for approximately 15min, so that the potatoes are soft.
2. Once the cooked potatoes are done we leave them 5 more minutes in the pot before taking them out.
3. Take them out and sauté with 2 tablespoons of butter and 1 glass of milk. When this mixture thickens, remove and transfer to a bowl, then crush them with a fork, as if you are making mashed potatoes.
4. Prepare 3 dishes with flour, egg, and breadcrumbs. Now take the potato portions and mold them into around shape, then pass them through the flour, then egg, and finally the breadcrumbs.

5. Raise the temperature of the fryer to 200º and put the balls in. When they are golden brown take them out and drain them on absorbent paper to remove excess oil.
6. To make the celery nest, clean the celery and julienne it, once cut, pass it through the flour and, with a strainer, remove the leftover flour and fry them, taking care that they do not burn.
7. Plate the fried celery and place the balls on top. As an accompaniment I add garlic, but it can be accompanied with any type of sauce. Also, the potato balls can be filled with any type of ingredient: such as bacon, peppers, onion, meat, or really anything you want! Though I often cook mine without stuffing.

28. Harness Croquettes

Ingredients

4 portions
- 1/2 Liter milk
- 40-45 g flour (all use)
- 60 ml (olive) oil
- The meat of exploitation
- Salt
- to taste nutmeg

------- Now we will have prepared:

- To wrap the croquettes.
- Abundant oil for frying in pan
- saucepan or fryer
- Breaded flour
- Bread crumbs
- 2 beaten eggs

Preparation

40 minutes

1. Put a pan or saucepan on the stove with the oil, add the flour and let it brown without burning. Gradually add the milk, letting it cook and bubble, then add the salt, nutmeg and meat that we will already have cut to our liking. Add more salt and let it thicken while bubbling, stirring along the way so that it does not stick. Pass it to a bowl or container and cover with transparent film glued to the

dough so that it does not crust, then let it cool in the refrigerator. Now you are ready to prepare or wrap the dough.

2. I do it with two spoons, taking portions of the dough and giving them a little shape before passing through the flour, egg, and breadcrumbs, I then leave them on a plate or dish.
3. And when they are all coated and we have the oil ready, we fry them and drain them well so that they are not oily. You can accompany them with salad, or with mayonnaise.

29. Uncle Pepe croquettes

Ingredients

10 portions
- 3 cans of tuna, or pickled tuna
- 1 onion
- 1 liter milk
- 4 tbsp flour
- olive oil (squirt to fry the onion)
- Salt
- bread crumbs
- 1 deep fryer full of hot oil

Preparation

50 minutes

1. First poke the onion.
2. Then add 4 tablespoons of flour.
3. Toast the flour a little and then add the pickled bonito with all its caldito.
4. Stir and slowly pour the milk until it begins to thicken the kissamel.
5. Test and salt to taste.
6. Allow to cool (a couple of hours minimum until the kissamel cooled).
7. Shape them up.
8. Beat a couple of eggs and coat the croquettes, then pass through the breadcrumbs, egg, and then breadcrumbs again.
9. Then with the fryer and very hot oil fry them.

30. Baked york cheese, egg and ham potatoes

Ingredients

- Potatoes
- Onion (optional)
- York ham
- Mozzarella cheese (preferably grated)
- Eggs
- Frying pan for potatoes
- Oven heat resistant casserole dish

Preparation

1. Peel and slice the potatoes.
2. Fry them a little, because otherwise they will be raw. They can be fried with a little onion to add flavor.
3. Put in the casserole dish: a layer of potatoes, a layer of ham, a layer of mozzarella cheese, another of potatoes, another of York, etc.
4. Put the casserole in the oven.
5. When the cheese has melted almost completely, take out the casserole and lay the eggs on top. Put back in the oven.
6. Leave in the oven for a couple more minutes, paying attention to see that the egg whites are cooked. Then take out of the oven and it is ready to eat!

31. Salmon in a bread crumb

The people in the north say "a fish roll says more than a thousand words". In the north, a world fish sandwich day was dedicated to the fish sandwich. We have a real appetite for fish sandwiches. They are quick to make and so delicious that everyone would like to have a second one! The fish is wrapped in bread dough and baked in the airfryer. Though in this recipe the bread is not cut open and stuffed, because the fish is already inside.. A filled salmon sandwich with sour cream and chives - what more could you want?

Ingredients for the bread

- 250 g Bread Mix
- 170ml water

- 60g linseed
- 160g Sunflower seeds
- 50g pumpkin seeds
- 1 1/2 tsp mustard
- 1 glass water
- some flour to work with

Preparation

1. Peel onions, then finely dice. Core the apple, cut into fine strips and then into small cubes. The salmon is also cut into cubes. Finely chop the mint, mix well with all remaining ingredients in a bowl, season with salt and pepper as needed.
2. The mass is then filled into a spherical shape and deep-frozen for 1 hour. Tip: you can also put small portions on baking paper and freeze.
3. For the dough, mix the flour with the water, knead for 10 minutes and let rest for 30 minutes. In the meantime, pulsate the grains in a blender or chop roughly. When the dough has doubled in size, it is again kneaded well and portioned into 12 equal parts. Now hammer one ball into the dough. Next, the fish sandwiches are dipped in water and then rolled in the grains.
4. Leave the salmon rolls at 55 ° C for 17 minutes, then bake at 160 ° C for 13 minutes. Tip: If you are not sure if the buns are really finished, you can test with a needle to see if they are hot inside.

The rolls can be served with a dip of sour cream and chives.

32. Kassler Sauerkraut Balls

Around the Kasseler or Kassler the myths entwine - where exactly did it come? Exactly who invented it is not clear. Of course, as electoral Berliners with our electoral Berlin city patriotism, we believe only one story, which is that of the Berlin butcher Cassel. Mr. Cassel had his butcher's shop on Potsdamer Strasse in Berlin Schöneberg and, one day, he put a pig's back in brine to make it last. You might have wished for a bit more glamor in the origin story, but often the greatest things happen without much fanfare! We have packed the classic combination of pancakes and sauerkraut in snack form, transforming every buffet on this planet into a gourmet temple. From Berlin with love!

Ingredients For The Dough

- 250 g Kasseler
- 200 g sauerkraut
- 1/2 pack of puff pastry

- 2 egg yolk
- mustard

Preparation

1. Dab the casserole dry, cut into cubes. Drain the sauerkraut a little using a sieve, this step is important, otherwise the balls are too moist and quickly soak the puff pastry.
2. Now lay out cling film on a board, then lay out a little sauerkraut, then the Kassler cubes and more sauerkraut. Now the film is beaten together, then firmly screwed. The balls have to be put in the freezer for one hour and the time in the freezer can vary, so that the puff pastry can be wrapped nicely around it
3. Cut the puff pastry into strips, beat each ball in 2 strips and place in the Airfryer baking dish. Mix 2 egg yolks with a little water and brush the balls with it. Bake at 160 ° C for 14 minutes, then crisp them at 185 ° C for 4 minutes. Serve the Kassler balls with mustard.

33. Sweet sweets from the airfryer

Pierogi like grandma, it comes with minced meat and sauerkraut. Today we will fill them with quark and dates. A simple pasta dough, filled, cooked, this is real manual work, so to speak. Baked in airfryer and ready to enjoy.

Ingredients For 23 Pieces
- 250 g Flour
- 1 egg
- 1/2 tsp oil
- 100ml water
- 160g Datteln
- 500g Quark
- 100 g sugar
- 1 1/2 tsp cinnamon

Preparation

1. Knead flour, water, oil, and egg into a homogenous dough, chill for 30 minutes. In the meantime, cut the dates into small pieces, let the quark drain briefly and mix with the dates.
2. Bring salted water to a boil in a saucepan. Knead the dough well again, roll out approx. 5 mm thick and cut into the desired size. Tip: You can use a glass for this. Put a spoonful of cottage cheese in the middle of the circles, fold half

together and squeeze with a fork. Put the raw dumplings in the water and cook for about 5-6 minutes.

3. Put the bacon in the Airfryer baking dish, fry at 160 ° C for 5 minutes. Add the pies and bake for 5 minutes, turn once and bake for another 5 minutes. Refine with a flake of butter and bake for 5 minutes at 190 ° C. Mix sugar and cinnamon, arrange the finished crunchy pierogi on a plate and sprinkle with sugar and cinnamon.

34. Green Shakshuka with the Airfryer baking pan

The dish, which probably originates from the North African region , comes from the airfryer today and is green instead of red. Spinach, eggs, and spicy feta cheese are then added - a real culinary delight!

Ingredients For 3-4 People
- 1/2 bunch spring onions
- 2 Red onions
- 2 Garlic cloves
- 1/2 bunch coriander
- 1/2 bunch parsley
- 3 kg spinach
- 4 tbsp olive oil
- eggs
- 80gfeta cheese
- Salt and pepper

Preparation

Cut the spring onions into thin rings, peel the garlic and finely dice. Finely chop coriander. Sort the spinach, wash and drain briefly.

Heat the oil in a pan and sauté the onions, garlic and spring onions. Add spinach. Put a lid on it and sauté briefly. Now everything goes into the baking mold of the Airfryer. Whisk eggs and spread on the spinach.

The baking pan now goes into the airfryer at 160 ° C for 15 minutes. Then sprinkle with feta cheese, parsley and cilantro and serve with a really good bread.

35. Avocado on toast with poached egg!

Is there anything better than fresh country bread, a ripe avocado, and a perfectly poached egg from the airfryer? That is the mission in this recipe. Of course, this also applies to bread. Made easy and fast.

Ingredients for 4 persons

- 1-2 loaves of country bread
- eggs
- 100 g spinach
- 3 mature avocados
- 100 g butter
- 1-2 tbsp vinegar
- Salt and pepper

Preparation

Slice the country bread into thick slices. Cut the avocado in half, hollow it out with a spoon, slice it into thin slices, and season with a little salt and pepper.

Now heat 1 liter of water and 1-2 tablespoons of vinegar in the Airfryer baking pan at 200 ° C. Beat the eggs in a cup and set aside. Roast the slices of bread with butter in the pan, then add leaf spinach.

When the water is hot, you can put the eggs into the water one at a time with a ladle and cook at 200 ° C for 3 minutes. Tip: Do only 2 eggs per run, otherwise it will be too tight in the baking pan and the eggs will stick together after cooking.

Now you can serve, first the spinach on the bread, then the avocado, and finally the 2 poached eggs on top. Add a little watercress for the spiciness, if necessary, then a little salt and pepper for seasoning.

36. A BREAD ROLL AND AN EGG

Simply smearing a roll and frying an egg is yesterday's news! Today everything comes together that belongs together: rolls, bacon, onion, and egg unite and it is damn delicious. So easy and so good!

Ingredients for 4 persons

- 4 whole-grain bread rolls
- 4 eggs
- 40g spring onions
- 8 slices bacon
- 50gbutter
- 80gcheese
- Salt and pepper

Preparation

1. Cut the rolls and hollow them out with the help of a spoon. Chop the spring onions, mix with the cheese, and season.
2. Spread buns with butter and cover with bacon, separate egg whites from yolks. Add the egg whites to the spring onion and cheese and, with a spoon, add them to the bread. Put the egg yolk on top.
3. Bake the rolls at 160 ° C for 10-12 minutes in the baking tray of the Airfryer. Tip: With a flake butter you can refine the buns again. To test whether your buns are even, you can use the wooden skewer trick. If it sticks when poked, give the bun another minute.

37. Cordon Bleu Balls

Cordon Bleu is an absolute classic! However, it is relatively complicated in its preparation. We imagined how cool it would be to be able to offer this dish as a snack. That this would be a real eye-catcher, goes without saying. So Jens has gone to the kitchen and tried a little. The result is this snack, which thanks to the Airfryer gets along without a fat bath and therefore can be enjoyed without a guilty conscience!

Ingredients for 12 servings
- 270g cooked ham
- 200 g Cheese (in one piece)
- 4 pork cutlets
- 3 eggs
- 100 g Flour
- 70gPanko
- Salt and pepper
- wooden skewers
- cranberries

Preparation

1. To prepare, cut the cheese into cubes and cut the ham into strips about as wide as the cheese cubes.
2. Chop the schnitzel flat with a meat mallet, season with salt & pepper and cut so that a cheese and ham cube can be rolled into it.
3. For breading, we recommend the mega practical breading street - so you are spared the usual mess, which often arises when breading. In one bowl add

panko, and in another the eggs, in the last the flour. Now put the balls first in the flour, then in the whisked eggs, and finally in the panko.

4. Now spray the balls with oil - for an optimal result, an oil sprayer should be used. Alternatively, the balls can be spread with a little liquid butter. Cook at 200 ° C for 13 minutes in the Airfryer.

38. Cheese ham pluck bread

This Zupfbrot is suitable for a variety of occasions: barbecue, birthday, cozy round with friends or family, as an appetizer or just as is. They always go down well! The preparation is easy and the ingredients are in every small supermarket. In less than an hour everything is ready and can be eaten immediately. A dish made for the Airfryer!

For The Dough
- 250ml milk
- 40gyeast
- 500g Flour
- 1 egg
- 70gbutter
- pinch of salt
- 20gsugar

Covering

- 150g cheese
- 180g cooked ham

For painting
- 100 g butter
- 1 clove of garlic

Preparation

1. Heat the milk in a saucepan and dissolve the yeast in it. Add the flour and other ingredients and mix everything into a homogenous dough. Leave in a warm place for 30 - 60 minutes.
2. Cut the cheese and ham into strips about 3cm wide. Heat the butter and mix with minced garlic, set aside.
3. Now knead the dough vigorously and roll it out. Cut into 10 equal strips, brush with garlic butter, top with cheese and ham and roll up. Put the finished rolls

into the back kit of the Airfryer and bake for 10 minutes at 160 ° C. Brush again with garlic butter and bake for another 5 minutes.

39. Green focaccia from the Philips Airfryer

Focaccia - an aromatic flatbread made from yeast dough, which even the Romans consumed abundantly and which counts as a forerunner for the world's most famous pizza! Traditionally, bread is topped with olive oil, salt, and possibly herbs before baking and was part of breakfast. Since then, it has become an independent meal, which is served in different variations, e.g. with olives, onions, or in a snail shape. Our intern Jens has come up with something special and prepared a green variant in the airfryer with parsley!

Ingredients for 1 focaccia

- 225g wheat flour
- 40gyeast
- 4 tbsp olive oil
- 2bunch parsley
- 200ml water
- 30gSun-dried tomatoes
- 40ggreen olives
- 40gblack olives
- 2 sprigs of rosemary
- Pinch of salt & sugar

Preparation

1. Preparation: Wash the parsley, finely chop and mix with the water. Sift flour and place in a bowl, chop rosemary, olives and dried tomatoes.
2. Now press the soaked parsley through a sieve and knead with the flour, tomatoes and olives to a homogeneous dough. Let it sit for 30 minutes.
3. Knead the dough again after the rest period and distribute in the baking tin of the Airfryer. Let it rest for another 10 minutes and then bake at 160 ° C for 18 minutes.

40. chicken tikka masala

Chicken Tikka Masala (also abbreviated as CTM) is a dish offered by many Indian restaurants within Europe and North America. It is composed of marinated chicken meat and a spicy tomato sauce, and actually originated in England. To give the chicken a special CTM taste, it is marinated in yoghurt and spices for several hours.

Although this dish is traditionally cooked in a pot, we have used baking mold of the Airfryer - and it worked well!

Our tip: briefly toast the spices in a pan, so you deepen the taste of your dish!

Ingredients for 3-4 people

- 400g Chicken breast fillet
- 200 g canned tomatoes
- 250ml Natural yoghurt
- 1 onion
- 2 Garlic cloves
- 1 teaspooncoriander seeds
- 1/2 tsp cinnamon
- 1 teaspoonpaprika
- 1 teaspoon turmeric
- 1 teaspoon curry spice
- 1 teaspoon mustard seeds
- 1 tbsp tomato paste
- Chili (or more, for those who like it hot)
- 30g fresh ginger
- 240g Basmati rice
- 1 bunch coriander

Preparation

1. Dice the chicken breast roughly and mix in a bowl with the yoghurt and place covered in the fridge for 4-6 hours or overnight.
2. Peel the ginger and onions and finely chop the tomatoes, onions, and ginger. Remove the seeds of the chili peppers and mince them and dice the garlic.
3. Mix the vegetables with the marinated chicken. Add tomato paste and spices and mix well again.
4. Now put the whole mass in the baking pan and cook everything at 180 ° C for about 25 minutes. Serve with basmati rice and cilantro, season if necessary.

41. Persian herbal frittata

Kuku Sabzi calls this a specialty from Iran and it has taken our office by storm! A true taste explosion, which makes use of numerous herbs. The eggs hold it all together. Just looking at the list of ingredients triggers screams of enthusiasm - at least for us. The best thing about this dish is that it's super fast to prepare. Simply chop the herbs in the FoodPro, and bake the omelette in the Airfryer. Only the onions and leeks / spring onions must be briefly simmered in a pan.

Our tip: Serve the Kuku Sabzi with some yoghurt and a simple salad and we swear to you, you will find yourself in the middle of 1001 Nights!

Ingredients for 3-4 people

- cooking oil
- 1 onion
- 1 Leeks / scallion
- big eggs
- 1 1/2 tsp salt
- 1 teaspoonbaking powder
- 1 teaspoonblack pepper
- 1/2 tsp Turmeric (optional)
- Coriander, bunch
- Dill, bunch
- Parsley, bunch

Preparation

Heat the oil in the pan and sauté the onions, leeks or spring onions until they are tender but have not taken on much color.

Mince the herbs in the FoodPro.

Exchange the knife for the dough knife and add eggs, salt, baking powder and, if necessary, turmeric. Mix.

Add everything to the baking tin of the Airfryer and bake at 170 ° C for 20 minutes.

42. Fried halloumi with asparagus salad

This dish is perfect for the summer. It does not take much time to prepare it. Especially in summer, this is an enormously important feature, because you want to spend as much as possible outdoors and not spend an eternity preparing food. It's also a light meal - so you will not fall into the infamous food coma after you've eaten it. And of course, it tastes amazingly good!

Our tip: use the Philips Party Kit for the preparation, because then the halloumi and asparagus can be cooked at the same time.

Ingredients

- 1 tbsp sesame oil

- 1 teaspoon honey
- 1/2 tsp garlic powder
- Salt and pepper
- 4 Halloumi slices - 150g
- 4 tbsp sesame oil
- 500g Asparagus, green
- olive oil
- salt and pepper
- Lemon abrasion, to taste
- 200 g cherry tomatoes
- Basil, fresh
- Capers, to taste

Preparation

1. Mix sesame oil, honey, garlic powder and salt & pepper. Brush the halloumi with the marinade and then roll it in the sesame.
2. Wash the asparagus, cut off the ends and halve them lengthways. Marinate with olive oil, salt, pepper and lemon.
3. Place the halloumi and asparagus in the airfryer. With the help of the Philips Party Kit both can be put together in the Garkorb. Cook at 180 ° C for 15 minutes. Take out the asparagus, turn the Halloumi and cook at 200 ° C for another 3 minutes in the Airfryer.
4. Serve the halloumi and asparagus with cherry tomatoes, capers, and basil!

43. Juicy Lemon Ricotta Cake with the Airfryer

. A good cake is of course tasty, but balanced. It does not overwhelm, but animates. A good cake is juicy and not dry, you do not want to choke on it! A good cake must also be visually pleasing. Finally, the consistency is crucial. This cake combines all these qualities and is so much fun.

Ingredients
- 115g Butter, unsalted & at room temperature
- 150g Powdered sugar, alternatively sugar
- 1 teaspoon vanilla extract
- 3 Eggs, big
- 3 tbsp lemon juice

- Lemon abrasion of a whole fruit
- 140g Flour
- 2 Tea spoons baking powder
- 250 g ricotta
- 60ml milk
- Natural yoghurt, optional
- Raspberry compote, optional

Preparation

1. Mix the butter with the sugar and vanilla extract until the mixture is pale and creamy.
2. Gradually add the eggs until they are mixed with the butter mass. Then add lemon juice and grated cheese, flour, baking powder, and ricotta and stir well. Finally, add the milk and stir again. The mass may look a bit lumpy, but that's fine.
3. Now pour the mixture into the baking tin of the Airfryer and bake at 160 ° C for 35-40 minutes. It is optional to serve with natural yoghurt and raspberry compote.
4. For the raspberry compote, simply boil frozen raspberries to create a slightly viscous mass.

44. French Onion Soup Grilled Cheese Sandwich

What happens when you introduce French onion soup and a classic of American sandwich culture - the Grilled Cheese Sandwich? Something magical, be aware of that. A snack, whose exuding fragrances have a beguiling effect on the unprepared. Distracted by the flavors that hang in the air, they will find you, come what may! And you will not get around to sharing your portion.

Our tip: use the grill pan for the Airfryer XXL to grill the sandwiches . That's the only way to get a nice even grill!

Ingredient

FOR 4 SANDWICHES

- 2-3onions
- 5 tbsp Butter & more to brush
- 1 tbsp olive oil
- 1 teaspoonthyme
- 1 teaspoonsugar

- Salt and pepper
- 3 tbsp beef broth
- 4 Slices of bread, big
- 200 Gruyère or Swiss mountain cheese

Preparation

1. Cut the onions into rings. Melt the butter in the pan, add the oil and fry the onions for 5 minutes.
2. Add salt, sugar, pepper, and thyme. Cover the pan and wait for everything to be evenly caramelized. Finally, add the broth and let it evaporate. Set aside.
3. Cut the bread into 4 equal, thick pieces and butter from the outside. Turnover and top with cheese, place the onions on top, then more cheese and finally the second slice of bread. Grill at 180 ° C for 7-8 minutes per side.

45. Bananas marble cake with the baking dish

Banana cakes are a firm favorite for all of us, and even cafes have now accepted this pastry as a classic. The classic version involves bananas, flour, sugar, eggs, and possibly a pinch of cinnamon. How about a portion of cocoa to turn our beloved banana cake into a marble cake? The final result? a juicy, chocolate banana marble cake!

Ingredients

- 3 ripe bananas
- 100 g honey
- 50g
- melted butter
- 130g yogurt
- 1 teaspoon vanilla extract
- 200 g Wheat flour or whole wheat grain
- 1 teaspoon baking powder
- 1 pinch of salt
- 1 teaspoon cinnamon
- 60g Sunflower seeds
- 20g cocoa

Preparation

1. The bananas are pounded (the Mini Food Processor is excellent for this!) And then creamed with honey, butter, yoghurt, and vanilla. Now add flour, baking powder, salt, and cinnamon and make a smooth dough. Stir the sunflower seeds (except 1 tbsp) evenly into the dough.
2. Grease the baking tin a little and cut the dough in half. Mix one half of the dough with the cocoa and alternately fill 2 tbsp white, then dark dough into the baking tin. Finally, whisk the dough roughly with a toothpick or knife to create a marbled pattern. Spread the remaining sunflower seeds on the cake and then bake at 170 ° C for 35-40 minutes.

46. Apple chips from the airfryer

Do you fancy fruity chips? Then these apples dried in the airfryer are just the thing for you! All that is needed is apples and a little cinnamon - that's it. If you do not use the apple slices immediately after cutting, you can use a few drops of lemon juice: this will stop the fresh apple slices browning. The snack kit is also very helpful as it prevents the very thinly cut discs from flying around. Well then, let's go!

Ingredients

- 2 apples
- 1/4 tsp cinnamon

Preparation

1. Wash the apples, remove the peels and cut the apples into 2mm thin slices using a kitchen slicer. Place the apple slices one at a time in the Airfryer. It is not bad if some slices touch each other - this is unavoidable with the amount we are making. Evenly spread some cinnamon over the apple slices. Put on the splash guard of the snack kit and bake the apple slices at 85 ° C for 1 hour.
2. After an hour, lift the splash guard with the help of the Snack Kit pliers and separate the chips - these stick together a little bit. Return the splash guard to the Airfryer tray and cook the chips for another 25 minutes. Now they should be as crisp as chips!

47. Vegetable chips with the snack kit

Ingredients

- 3 small potatoes
- 1.2 sweet potato
- beetroot, uncooked
- 2-3 carrots

- 2 tbsp Liquid honey
- 1 tbsp hot mustard
- 2 tbsp oil
- 1 teaspoon vinegar
- Salt pepper

Preparation

1. Cut the potatoes and sweet potato into thin slices (about 2mm) and cover with water for at least 10 minutes in a deep bowl to allow the starch to escape. Also, cut the beetroot and carrots into thin slices. After 10 minutes lay the potatoes on a tea towel and cover with a second cloth, lightly pat dry.
2. Mix honey, mustard, oil, vinegar, salt, and pepper in a small bowl until smooth. Put all the vegetable slices in a large bowl and mix with the honey and mustard mixture. To get crispy chips, we recommend baking only half of the total amount in the airfryer at 150 ° C for 25-30 minutes with the splash guard. It is important to shake the chips every 10 minutes to make them evenly crisp.
3. Allow to cool for a few minutes after baking, because only then will they get our beloved chip consistency.

48. Three quiche in the Airfryer baking pan

Almost everyone likes to eat quiche, but spending hours in the kitchen to first knead the dough, then prepare the filling, and then wait for it to bake: no one loves this. With the help of the Airfryer and its practical baking pan, you can make a tasty quiche in no time at all. The basic recipe can be applied to any type of quiche, namely featuring eggs, sour cream, cheese, pepper, and salt. With the dough, we have made it very easy and will cook in the baking pan with only standard puff pastry ingredients needed. The filling is mixed together in a jiffy - and your quiche is ready!

Ingredient

Filling Basic Recipe

- 3 eggs
- 1 cup Sour cream (200g)
- 80g grated cheese (eg Gouda or Emmental)
- salt and pepper

For The Quiche Lorraine

- 2 Onions, chopped small
- 125g bacon

- 1.2Leek, cut into rings
- 1 puff pastry
- salt and pepper
- 20ggrated cheese

For The Spinach Blue Chicken Quiche

- 1 Onion, chopped small
- 250 g spinach
- 200 g Blue cheese
- 50gpine nuts
- 1 puff pastry
- salt and pepper
- 20ggrated cheese

For The Asparagus And Serrano Quiche

- 1 Onion, chopped small
- 400g white or green asparagus
- 50gSerrano ham
- 1 puff pastry
- salt and pepper
- 20ggrated cheese

Preparation

1. In a bowl whisk the eggs with sour cream and then stir in grated cheese. Season with salt and pepper.
2. For the Quiche Lorraine: fry the onions and bacon in a pan, allow to cool and add to the filling. Add the leek rings and season with salt and pepper.

For the spinach and blue chicken quiche: Fry the onions in a pan, add the spinach and sauté for 5 minutes. Allow the spinach and onion mixture to cool slightly, add to the filling and mix well. Break the blue cheese into large pieces and place in the filling.

For the asparagus-serrano quiche: Fry the onions in a pan, allow to cool and stir into the filling. Peel the asparagus, cut into 2-3 cm long pieces and add to the egg mass. Coarsely grate the Serrano ham and fold it in. Season with salt and pepper.

Place the puff pastry in the pan and make sure there is enough dough around the edges. Excess dough can easily be cut off. Pour the filling over the puff pastry and either gently squeeze or roll the edges of the dough so that the quiche crust is even.

Add the filling and sprinkle with the rest of the cheese. Bake the quiches in the airfryer for 25-30 minutes at 180 ° C (the asparagus quiche takes a little longer due to the water in the asparagus: we recommend 35-40 minutes at 160 ° C). Let each quiche cool for 10 minutes and serve.

49. Stuffed Mediterranean peppers with the party kit

Whoever invented stuffed peppers, he or she was nothing short of a genius. A genius, because it could not be easier. A genius, because it is actually obvious to add paprika - and yet nobody did it before. Anyway, let's give that somebody a little tribute with this dish. The ingenious thing about this dish is that you can make it completely in the Airfryer! All it takes is the handy Philips Party Kit for the Airfryer XXL . Simply prepare peppers and garnish on the day to save time and effort. This recipe is at least as ingenious as the invention of stuffed peppers themselves.

Ingredients for 2 persons
- about 175gminced meat
- 3-4red peppers
- 1 Spring onion, chopped
- Garlic cloves, pressed
- 1 teaspoonsmoked paprika
- 1 teaspoonchilli flakes
- about 30gSoft cheese, e.g. feta
- 2-3Sweet potatoes, big
- 1 bag Sweet potato fries (optional)
- 100 g Gouda, grated
- Salt and pepper

Preparation

1. Remove the stalk of the pepper and cut a lid along it with a knife. Remove the core and seeds.
2. Mix the mince meat, spring onions, garlic, paprika, chilli flakes, and feta cheese. Season with salt and pepper and fill the peppers with this mix. Put the cheese on top and the sweet potato fries in the airfryer. Thanks to the basket separator,the party kit fits both in together. Cook at 180 ° C for 13-15 minutes - done!

50. Pizza Flammkuchen Style from the Airfryer

We have already made tarte flambée, but not yet in the airfryer. We just could not leave it and had to find out how the Pizza Kit for the Airfryer XXL performs. The result has absolutely convinced us! We used a yeast mix for the dough, so the result is something of an onion cake. We have worked with yeast dough, but many know the Flammkuchen Alsatian style for its wafer-thin, very crispy dough. Therefore we have included the information to make both variants.

For The Yeast Dough

Ingredient

- 300g Flour
- pinch of sugar
- pinch of salt
- 3 tbsp oil
- 150ml water
- 1 Pck. Dry yeast

Alsatian dough

- 220g Flour
- 3 tbsp olive oil
- 1 egg yolk
- 1/2 tsp salt
- 100ml Water, warm

For Covering

- 2small onions, red
- 125g bacon
- Handful of chives
- 2Garlic cloves
- 1 Cup of sour cream
- 1 Mug creme fraiche
- Salt and pepper
- 1 spring onion

Preparation

1. For the dough, dissolve the yeast in 50 ml of water and add a pinch of sugar. In a bowl, mix the flour, pinch of salt, oil, and yeast water into a smooth dough. Let it sit for 30 minutes. Mix ALTERNATIVE flour, 2 tablespoons of olive oil, egg yolk, salt, and water to a smooth dough. Spread dough ball with remaining oil and let it rest in foil for 30 minutes at room temperature.
2. Now the dough can be rolled out. For the pizza kit it should have a 26cm diameter.

3. Crème fraiche, sour cream, garlic (pressed) and stir the chives. Season with salt & pepper and distribute about 3 tablespoons on a rolled out flat bread. Cover with bacon cubes and onion. Bake at 200 ° C for 10 minutes.

51. Beef and Onion BBQ Pizza from the Airfryer

Søren has the favor of the moment - the pizza kit for the Philips Airfryer XXL is here - and grabbed his favorite pizza prepared. It is not known where he got the recipe from, but it can be assumed it was the result of years of trying it out. The composition may seem a bit strange, but you should not let it unsettle you. Trust the man, Søren knows what's good!

Ingredients

FOR 1 PIZZA
- Pizza dough
- 60gminced meat
- 3 tbsp sieved tomatoes
- 1 clove of garlic
- 1 tbsp Bbq sauce
- 1 small red onion
- Jalapeños, at will
- 1 teaspoonchilli flakes
- 1.2Mozzarella
- Cheddar, at will
- Parmesan, at will

Preparation

1. Roll out the dough thinly and place on the pizza kit.
2. For the tomato sauce, combine tomatoes, BBQ sauce, crushed garlic, and chili flakes. Spread on the dough and top with the other ingredients.
3. Bake at 200 ° C for 6 minutes. If you like it darker then 7 - 8 minutes.

52. Cheese sticks from the Philips Airfryer

An integral part of the classic party snacks: the cheese bar. We'll show you how to prepare it in no time using the airfryer. Since we generally believe that Parmesan never spoils, we have upgraded our cheese sticks with some Parmesan. This basic recipe can be refined or modified at will and taste.

Ingredient

FOR 3-4 PEOPLE

- 1 pack puff pastry
- 2 tbsp tomato paste
- 100 g Gouda, grated
- 50g Parmesan, grated
- 1 egg
- 1 Shot of milk
- =Sesame to garnish

Preparation

1. Roll out the puff pastry and spread with the tomato paste. Next spread the Parmesan on the dough and then the Gouda. Press lightly so that not so much cheese is "lost" when turning.
2. Now cut the dough with a knife into 1 cm thick strips. Pick up both ends and twist like a cord (both ends in the opposite direction). To fit in the airfryer, divide the dough strands in the middle.
3. Whisk the egg and milk and brush sticks with it. So they get a nice appetizing color while baking and the sesame seeds are also much crispier! Sprinkle with sesame seeds and bake at 180 ° C for 8 minutes in the airfryer.

53. Baltic Garlic Bread Sticks With Yogurt Dip

Garlic bread, baguette or sticks are a popular snack no matter what name you use. I spent some time in the northernmost of the three Baltic States and learned to appreciate the garlic bread there very much. Küüslauguleivad , as they are called in Estonia, is an elementary part of the snack and bar culture there. Meeting with some friends in the pub in the evening, you can be sure too see garlic bread on the table. The special thing is that only black bread is used for it. We know garlic bread rather than baguette or another white bread. We did it with a gray mixed bread. An authentic experience that you get only with black bread! Traditionally a dip of garlic mayonnaise or hapukoor (sour cream) is served alongside, we made a yoghurt dip with parsley.

Ingredients

FOR 3-4 PEOPLE

- 1 Loaf of bread, if possible black
- 6 tbsp olive oil
- 2-3 Garlic cloves, pressed
- 1 tbsp garlic powder
- FOR THE DIP

- 250 g Yogurt / cottage cheese
- 1 Handful of parsley
- 1 Shot of olive oil
- Salt and pepper
- Lemon, optional

Preparation

1. Cut the bread into finger-sized fries. Optionally, you can roast the bread at 180 ° for about 8 minutes before.
2. In the meantime, the garlic can be squeezed into the olive oil and garlic powder added. Mix well and add a little salt.
3. Now to the dip. To do this, mix the yoghurt / quark with the parsley, a dash of olive oil and salt and pepper.
4. Spread the crispy bread chips generously with the garlic oil and pour into the airfryer for 10 minutes at 180 ° C - done.

54. Muzen from the Airfryer

One of the highlights of the 5th season is guaranteed: the Muzen! The almond-shaped, butter biscuit-like pastry is traditionally eaten at Festelovend a.k.a Carnival. Of course, we should not miss it - even if this carnival in the east of Germany is not celebrated. The preparation is very simple and the dough bakes well in an Airfryer - so you can save yourself the bath in the frying fat! Helau & Alaaf!

Ingredients

FOR ABOUT 25 PIECES

- 325g Flour
- 1 1/2 tsp baking powder
- 100 g sugar
- 2 eggs
- 1 pinch of salt
- 100 g soft butter / margarine

Preparation

1. Mix the flour and baking powder together in a bowl. Add the other ingredients and mix well. It's best to use your hands and knead the dough beautifully.

2. Roll the dough into small, almond-like shapes. The smaller you roll the almonds, the more coins you get out. Lay out the Airfryer with baking paper and bake the coins for 10 minutes at 200 ° C.
3. Optionally, you can coat the finished Muzen with liquid butter and roll in sugar. After all, it's Carnival and Muzen are not eaten every day!

55. Roasted almonds from the airfryer

Roasted almonds do not just have to be at Christmas, because they turn out to be very, very good. They are easy to prepare and it does not take much effort. The taste is just almonds - so by itself already very delicious! Add a little honey to it and some coarse sea salt and you've conjured up a snack that you wish you will never run out of!

Ingredients

FOR 4 PEOPLE
- about 240galmonds
- 1 teaspooncoarse salt
- 1 teaspoonhoney

Preparation

1. Let the almonds soak overnight. Rinse thoroughly the next morning.
2. Mix the washed almonds well with the honey, salt and a little olive oil and place in the Airfryer at 200 ° C for 15 minutes.
3. drizzle witholive oil

56. Avocado fries from the airfryer

A party snack that will please many. Avocado fries are super yummy, can made fast and do not need a long ingredient list. The breading can be designed according to taste and makes this snack very diverse. Perfect for a cozy TV evening or when friends come to visit.

Ingredients

FOR 3-4 PEOPLE
- 2 avocados
- Pankomehl
- 1 teaspoonpaprika
- 1 teaspoonsalt
- 2 eggs
- oil

Preparation

1. Halve the avocados, detach from the core and peel. Cut into strips.
2. Whisk the eggs for the breading and mix the panko with the salt and paprika powder. Roll the avocado strips in the egg and then in the breadcrumbs. Sprinkle with oil and place in the Airfryer at 200 ° C for 8 minutes.

57 Banana Bread Waffles with the Philips Airfryer

Valentine's Day is approaching! The perfect time to please someone. It does not have to be a big effort, it depends mainly on the gesture! With these delicious waffles, this can be done quickly. A sweet breakfast that will be remembered for a long time (and that will surely be requested again)!

Ingredients

FOR 4 SERVINGS

- 250 g Flour
- 1 teaspoonbaking powder
- 1/2 tsp salt
- 115g butter
- 50gsugar
- 1 egg
- 1 egg yolk
- 60gSour cream / sour cream
- 1 teaspoonvanilla extract
- 3ripe bananas, crushed
- Maple syrup to serve

Preparation

1. In a bowl, mix the melted butter, sugar, egg, egg yolk, sour cream, and vanilla extract. Then add the three crushed bananas.
2. Gradually add the flour and baking soda until everything is well connected. Fill the waffle dish with dough and place in the Airfryer at 160 ° C for 14 minutes.

58. Raclette in the airfryer

Raclette - a classic. Melted cheese in combination with all sorts of side dishes such as potatoes, peppers, onions, mushrooms, pickled cucumbers, herbs, quark and delicious baguettes? Well that sounds good! On New Year's Eve, many Germans eat this popular variation of cheese fondue and we understand why. We have come up with a recipe for you that makes raclette with the Airfryer possible - so you do not have to dig a dusty raclette oven from the cellar and clean it up after the festivities. Instead, you can sit comfortably with your family at the table and use the Airfryer to make your stuffed potatoes - and whatever else you like - baked with cheese. Like the raclette!

Ingredients

FOR 4 PEOPLE
- 1 kgbig potatoes, cooked
- 500g raclette cheese
- 200 g mushrooms
- 2 Red onions
- 2 paprika
- 200 g Cherry tomatoes
- Herb quark
- Bread to serve
- Salt and pepper

Preparation

Halve the potatoes and hollow them out with a spoon (the potato interior can be used as a side dish for a potato salad, for example). Dice onions, peppers and mushrooms and put them in bowls. Halve the cherry tomatoes and cut the raclette cheese so that one slice fits on one potato half.

Fill the potato halves with some vegetables and then cover with a cheese slice. Cook in the Airfryer at 180 ° C for 6-8 minutes until the cheese has melted. Depending on how crusty you like your cheese, you can cook the potatoes after 6 minutes again for 2 minutes at 200 ° C.

Season with salt and pepper and serve with bread, herb quark and your favorite raclette side dishes.

59 Stuffed mushrooms from the airfryer

Stuffed mushrooms are very tasty - especially if the filling is based on ricotta and also includes dried tomatoes, red onions, and fresh parsley. These mushrooms are a taste experience - and making them in the Airfryer means less fat!

Ingredients

- big mushrooms
- 1 Red onion
- 2 Garlic cloves
- 70g Sun-dried tomatoes
- 250 g ricotta
- 1 tbsp olive oil
- 3 thyme sprigs
- fresh Parmesan
- parsley
- salt and pepper

Preparation

Wash the mushrooms and cut out the stalks. Sauté the leftover minced meat, diced onion, and finely chopped garlic in olive oil.

Finely chop the dried tomatoes and parsley and add to the pan. Poke the thyme into the mixture and mix everything with the ricotta. Season with salt and pepper and then fill in the mushrooms. Grate the fresh Parmesan cheese over the mushrooms and cook in the Airfryer at 180 ° C for 8 minutes.

Serve with Parmesan.

60. Hot chestnuts from the airfryer

Christmas markets - who does not love them? With roasted almonds, mulled wine and raclette cheese, we like to enjoy these small, festively decorated stalls. And what is missing in this delicious listing? Very clear: hot chestnuts! Sweet chestnuts are so delicious and we have good news for you: you can prepare them in your Airfryer!

Ingredients

- 200ml water
- 500g chestnuts

Preparation

1. Carve the chestnuts like a cross. Pour the water into the fat drip tray of the Airfryer and place the chestnuts in the Garkorb. Cook at 200 ° C for 14 minutes and serve hot!

61. Burnt almonds from the airfryer

Crunchy, sweet almonds are part of the Christmas market, just like balls on the Christmas tree. If you like them fresh and crunchy at home, you should definitely try this simple and quick recipe. You'll be surprised that your Airfryer makes the best burnt almonds you've ever eaten!

ingredients for 4 persons
- 400g almonds
- 160ml
- water
- 200 g Brown sugar
- 2 tbsp cinnamon

Preparation

1. Boil the sugar, water and cinnamon in a pot while stirring with a wooden spoon all the time. Stir in the almonds for a minimum of 2-3 minutes, stirring until the water has boiled over and the sugar becomes crumbly. Please make sure that the sugar does not burn.

2. Put the almonds in a layer on baking paper in the airfryer. Allow to dry at 160 ° C for 10 minutes. Put the almonds on a plate and allow to cool to make them crispy.

62 Wine pears in dressing gown

This sweet temptation is an absolute dream! The pears are cooked with cinnamon and aniseed stars in red wine and thus take on an indescribable aroma. Finally wrapped with puff pastry and baked in the Philips Airfryer. Simple and delicious! We recommend vanilla ice cream or sauce to accompany them.

Ingredients for 4 persons
- pears
- 1 bottle of red wine
- 2 cinnamon sticks

- Anise stars
- 1 Pack of puff pastry
- 1 egg yolk

Preparation

1. Put the red wine in a pot. Peel the pears and place in the red wine. Simmer for 60 minutes
2. Strip the puff pastry and wrap the pears with it. Brush with the yolk. Lay out the basket with baking paper and place in the Airfryer at 180 ° C for 12 minutes - done!

63 Roast beef with potato gratin and Bernaise sauce

Roast beef with potato gratin with sauce Bernaise - perfect for a cozy evening! Matthias came up with this feel-good dish as the main course for his Christmas meal, but it turns out that every evening demands something special! Everything except the sauce can be prepared in the Airfryer - so it does not even have to be cooked for hours! The quantities are estimated, as the chef usually cooks by eye. It should be enough for 4 people.

Ingredients

For The Roast Beef

- about 1.4 kg roast beef
- 5 tbsp mustard
- Salt pepper
- fresh thyme
- oil

For The Gratin

- about 5 potatoes
- 2 egg yolks
- 200ml cream
- 1 Pinch of nutmeg
- Salt and pepper
- 1 clove of garlic
- Parmesan
- Butter for greasing
- rosemary

For The Sauce
- 1 shallot
- egg yolks
- 1 teaspoon vinegar
- salt
- 2 Tea spoons water
- 125g Butter, melted

PREPARATION

1. Spread roast beef with mustard and season with salt and pepper. Add a few strands of fresh thyme and some oil to the airfryer. The meat gets 2 courses of cooking. First for 12 minutes at 200 ° C and then for 20 minutes at 180 ° C.
2. In the meantime, the potatoes can be peeled and sliced into slices with a planer.
3. Now mix 2 egg yolks with cream, nutmeg, salt, pepper, garlic, and Parmesan cheese. Grease the shape for the gratin with a piece of butter and fill it with the potatoes and the sauce. Add parmesan and some rosemary on top.
4. When finished, wrap the meat in aluminum foil with a piece of butter and let it rest.
5. Stir in the potato gratin at 180 ° C with some water in the bottom for 20 minutes in the airfryer.
6. Now the sauce Bernaise can be prepared. Add a shallot, 3 egg yolks, vinegar, water, and salt to a Food Processor. Slowly but evenly add melted butter until a slightly thick consistency is reached. Arrange and enjoy everything!

64   Goat cheese tartlets with figs, salad & pistachios

These little tartlets - or tartlets - not only make a stunning appetizer, but also make a great snack in between meals or evenings with friends! They are hearty and make a great contrast with the figs. The creamy consistency of the tartlets is perfectly complemented by the crisp and fresh salad. We are totally thrilled - Matthias has earned a pat on the back!

Ingredients

FOR 4 TARTLETS
- 2 tbsp Pistachios, chopped
- 120g Fresh cheese rolls
- 30gcream cheese
- Salt and pepper

- 1/2 tsp bread crumbs
- 2 tbsp whipped cream
- 1 tbsp Butter, melted
- Leaves filo pastry
- Stems thyme
- 150g salad

For the dressing

- Stalks dill
- 4 tbsp olive oil
- 1 teaspoonhoney
- 4 tbsp balsamic
- figs

Preparation

1. Stir cream cheese with egg, breadcrumbs, cream, salt, and pepper.
2. For 4 tartlets, cut 12 circles larger than the shape you use for baking.
3. Put a filo pastry circle in the bottom of a cake pan and butter. Repeat twice so that a total of 3 slices are on top of each other in the shape and form the bottom. Now fill with 2 tablespoons of cream cheese and top with 3 slices of goat's cheese. Garnish with thyme and brew for 10 minutes at 180 ° C in the Airfryer.
4. For the salad, mix the ingredients for the dressing together. Serve the salad with the figs next to the tartlets and drizzle with dressing.

65 Baked apple from the airfryer

An absolute classic at Christmas time, quasi the pop star of winter-Christmas desserts. Legend has it that there are even poems about him:

Children, come and guess what's roasting in the oven! Hear how it bangs and hisses. Soon he is served up, the corner, the apple, the top, the cap, the yellow-red apple.

Kids, run faster, bring a dish, bring a fork! Lock the beak for the tip, the apple, the top, the cap, the golden apple!

They blow and blow, they look and swallow, they click and taste, they lick and lick the tip, the apple, the top, the cap, the crunchy apple.

More does not have to be said!

FOR 4 PEOPLE

Ingredients

- apples
- 30g raisins
- 40g chopped hazelnuts
- 2 tbsp honey
- 1/2 tsp cinnamon
- vanilla extract

Preparation

1. Core the apples. Mix raisins, hazelnuts, honey, cinnamon, and vanilla extract and fill the apples with this mix.
2. Cook at 180 ° C for 10 minutes in the airfryer.

66 Rack of lamb with herb crust from the airfryer

Are you looking for a special recipe that fits well into a Christmas menu, for example: festive lamb crusted in herb crust, bedded on beetroot and potato puree and garnished with Parmesanchips? Does not that sound tempting? Exactly, we thought so too! You do not eat lamb dishes every day, and with a refined herbal and almond crust, they taste particularly spicy and tasty.

FOR 3-4 PEOPLE

Ingredients

- Rack of lamb, pre-cut
- 1 tbsp olive oil
- 1 clove of garlic
- salt and pepper
- 1 tbsp fresh rosemary, finely chopped
- 1 tbsp dried thyme
- 40gButter, melted
- 20g Panko breadcrumbs
- 50gAlmonds, chopped
- salt and pepper

For the side dishes

- 500g beetroot, cooked (+ 3 tbsp beetroot juice)
- 800g potatoes
- 50gbutter
- salt and pepper

- 1 piece of nutmeg
- 3 tbsp grated Parmesan
- fresh parsley, chopped

Preparation

1. Boil water in a large pot. Peel the potatoes and cook with the beetroot for about 30 minutes until the potatoes are tender. Add the butter and work with a potato masher until the puree is creamy. Season with nutmeg, salt and pepper.
2. Now marinate the rack of lamb. Brush with olive oil, season with salt and pepper and sprinkle with garlic. To prepare the herb breadcrumbs: mix the butter, rosemary, thyme, panko breadcrumbs, salt and pepper, and spread on the meat. Place on grill pan of the Airfryer and cook at 200 ° C for 10 minutes.
3. Melt the Parmesan in the Airfryer baking pan and allow to cool. Break into small pieces.
4. Arrange some puree on a plate and lay the meat on it. Then garnish with Parmesan asparagus and fresh parsley.

67 Spicy carrots from the airfryer

This dish is something different: spicy carrots paired with almonds and cranberries. And then a special spice is added to give the whole thing a unique taste: Ras el-Hanout. This spice mix originates from North Africa and consists of ginger, caraway, coriander, chili, paprika, cinnamon, allspice, and pepper. Does that not sound delicious? Lemon juice and skin give the carrots extra freshness - a side dish dream with aroma and bite!

Ingredients

FOR 4 PEOPLE
- 500g carrots
- ½ Lemon, juice and peel
- 1 Garlic clove, finely chopped
- 2 tbsp olive oil
- 1 teaspoonRas el-Hanout
- 1 prs Harissa
- salt and pepper
- 70gdried cranberries

- 30g planed almonds
- Spring onions for garnish
- Lemon slices to serve

Preparation

1. Peel and halve the carrots. Mix with olive oil, garlic cloves, Ras el-Hanout, Harissa, lemon juice and peel and salt and pepper. Cook in the Airfryer at 180 °C for 15 minutes.
2. Mix with cranberries and almonds. Finally serve with a little chopped spring onion and lemon wedges.

68   Beetroot carpaccio with pistachio crisp

A salad that is wonderfully easy to prepare in the Airfryer! Fine beetroot slices served with spicy goat's cheese and pistachio crisp. The flavors complement each other perfectly in this combination and are also ideal for festive occasions such as the Christmas season.

FOR 4 PEOPLE

Ingredients

- 500g Beetroot (cooked)
- 60g pistachios
- 2 tbsp honey
- 150g Goat cheese
- Salt pepper
- 1 teaspoon dried thyme
- Chives (optional)

Preparation

1. Chop the pistachios and mix with honey. Spread the baking tin with baking paper and spread the pistachio mass on top. Bake at 180 °C for 4 minutes and then at 200 °C for 2 minutes. Allow to cool.
2. Cut the red beets into thin slices and arrange on a plate.
3. Stir creamy goat cheese with salt, pepper, and thyme until creamy and spread on the beetroot. Sprinkle with the pistachio crisp and enjoy.

Panettone from the Airfryer

The Italian cuisine is especially loved in this country, but rather less associated with Christmas. The Italians have great food for the festive season, such as Panettone. This cake has its origins in Milan. According to legend, it was created out of necessity by a kitchen boy named Toni for his Lombard master, who was holding a sumptuous feast with other princes. Another dessert was planned, but because of the chef's carelessness was (rumors about the reason for this vary) burned in the oven. Toni's creation was so well received that the Pan di Toni (= Bread of Toni) became an integral part of Lombard's Christmas tradition. With your Airfryer you can now prepare Toni's gift for the Christmas season.

Ingredients

FOR 1 CAKE
- 200ml lukewarm milk
- Cubes of fresh yeast
- 100 g sugar
- 400g Flour
- 2 Vanilla pods, alternatively extract can be used
- 1 pinch of salt
- 2 egg yolks
- 100 g Butter (soft)
- 1 teaspoonlemon zest
- 60gCranberries
- 80gChocolate chips (bittersweet)
- 60gcandied peel
- 1 tbsp butter for brushing

Preparation

1. Mix the lukewarm milk with the yeast and 20g of sugar and set aside for 15 minutes.
2. Then add the rest of the sugar, flour, vanilla pulp, pinch of salt, egg yolks, butter and lemon juice and mix well. Rest in a warm place for at least 1.5 hours. The dough should have approximately doubled.
3. Now you can add cranberries, chocolate chips and the orange paste to the dough. Mix everything well so that it is evenly distributed. Let rest for another 40 minutes.

4. The dough can be baked either in the baking mold of the Airfryer at 160 ° C for 25 minutes or in smaller molds. We have made some of baking paper and kitchen yarn, because Panettone is traditionally baked in a similar mold.

70 Coq au vin from the airfryer

A dish from the haute cuisine of our dear neighbors for the Philips Airfryer: coq au vin. For those who do not know it: this is a French national dish, with vegetables and chicken braised in wine until a hearty and very tasty stew is produced. We have adapted this original Burgundy dish for the airfryer, so this delicacy can be prepared even if you do not have half the day for cooking. The result remains true to the original, so it fits well on festive occasions!

Ingredients

FOR 4 PEOPLE
- shallots
- 1 spring onion
- carrots
- 150ml chicken stock
- 150ml strong red wine
- 1 teaspoonPaprika powder (Rosenschaft & Edelsüß)
- 2Garlic cloves
- about 300gChicken (fillet or leg)
- Pepper and salt
- thyme
- 1-2Branches of fresh rosemary
- 1 Lemon peel (abrasion)
- 3 tbsp olive oil

Preparation

1. For the marinade, mince a carrot, spring onion, shallot, and garlic. Put this all in a bowl and add the wine, chicken stock, paprika, thyme, and rosemary (fresh if possible) as well as the lemon. Mix with the chicken and set aside for at least 30 minutes.

2. Chop the remaining carrots, shallots and garlic and sauté for 5 minutes at 180 ° C in the baking dish of the Airfryer with a little olive oil.
3. Then put the chicken drumsticks on top and put the contents of the bowl in the baking dish. Stir for 30 minutes at 140 ° C. If chicken drumsticks are used, turn them once after 15 minutes.
4. Serve on a deep plate. Potato dumplings or baked potatoes are excellent as a side dish. The latter can simply be prepared in the Airfryer: pour a little water into it and cook at 180 ° C for 30 minutes.

71 Baked gorgonzola pears from the airfryer

This dish is perfect as a warm starter in the cold season. In a sense, the warmth of Italy is being imported onto the plates, as the Gorgonzola and Porchetta are two of the main players in this recipe. However, that extra something makes the dressing for the chicory leaves. The tarragon gives the whole thing a festive touch, so that makes this warm salad also excellent as a starter for a Christmas dinner. But be warned, when a meal begins, the expectations for the following courses will be increased!

Ingredients

For The Salad
- 2 chicory piston
- 50gHazelnuts, roughly chopped
- 1 tbsp olive oil
- 2big ripe pears
- 100 g Gorgonzola
- 100 g Porchetta
- 2Slices of toasted bread
- 1 tbsp butter
- lemon juice

For The Dressing
- 3 tbsp olive oil
- 2 Tea spoons lemon juice
- 2 Tea spoons honey
- 1 tbsp Tarragon (or 1 bunch of chervil)
- Salt pepper
- 1 small pear

Preparation

1. Put the whole hazelnuts in the basket of the Airfryer. Brush the grill on top and the two slices of toast with the butter - this results in crispy croutons. Roast everything at 180 ° C for 7 minutes. Then roughly chop the hazelnuts and dice the toast. Put both aside - we'll need them for garnishing later.

2. Next, peel the two large pears, cut in half and remove their cores. Brush the pear halves with lemon juice as this acid prevents discoloration. Now just put the gorgonzola in the cavity and wrap everything with the porchetta. Cook at 160 ° C for 10 minutes in the baking pan.

3. For the dressing, peel the small pear, remove it from the core and cut into large pieces. Puree with the honey, olive oil, tarragon, lemon juice, salt and pepper in a food processor.

4. Wash the chicory and free it from its stalk. Cut into pieces and place on a plate. Drizzle on dressing and place a gorgonzola bulb wrapped in porchetta atop it. Garnish with roasted hazelnuts and croutons - ready!

72 Balsamic Brussels sprouts from the airfryer

A wonderfully simple dish with seasonal ingredients for the dingy autumn! Brussels sprouts, which get a very special touch from the balsamic vinegar, with deliciously aromatic baked potatoes and a simple herb quark. Less is sometimes more - this recipe is impressive proof!

Ingredients

FOR 4 PEOPLE
- 2 handfuls basil
  - 250 gSpeisequark
- 1 teaspoonolive oil
- Pepper and salt
- 4 potatoes
- 500gBrussel sprouts
- 1 tbsp olive oil
- 1 tbsp balsamic

Preparation

1. Put some water in the bottom of the Airfryer and put the 4 potatoes in the basket. Bake at 180 ° C for 30 minutes.
2. Add basil, olive oil, salt and pepper to the quark and mix well.

3. Halve the Brussels sprouts and marinate with olive oil, balsamic vinegar, salt and pepper. Place in the Airfryer at 180 ° C for 12 minutes.
4. Halve the baked potatoes, fill with the quark and add the Brussels sprouts - done!

73 Eggplant salad from the airfryer

That the Philips Airfryer can also produce salad, is proven with this latest recipe! Especially in autumn, hot salads have their own charm, and are extremely easy to make! Judith made this salad secretly, but since it tasted exceptionally good, we do not want to keep it from you.

Ingredients

FOR 2-3 PERSONS
- 1 aubergine
- 1 Red onion
- 2 Garlic cloves
- 1 tbsp olive oil
- 1 tbsp Sesame seeds
- Salt & pepper (to taste)
- 2 tbsp Tahini
- Lemon (juice)
- 1 pomegranate
- 1 Handful of mint
- Handful of parsley

Preparation

1. Wash the eggplant and cut into small cubes. Also chop the onion and garlic. Put everything in a bowl and mix with olive oil, salt, pepper and sesame seeds. Cook at 180 ° C for 12 minutes in the Airfryer.
2. In the meantime, the pomegranate can be cut open and freed from its kernels. Roughly chop mint and parsley. Mix the tahini sauce with lemon juice, salt and pepper.
3. Mix the aubergine from the airfryer with parsley, mint and pomegranate, serve the tahini sauce as a dip - done!

74 Nutty goat's cheese from the airfryer

Spicy, soft goat cheese tastes good to many of us. And as everyone knows, walnuts, honey and thyme are great with it. So we decided to bake goat's cheese slices with a mixture of these three ingredients in the airfryer - but only for a very short time, otherwise the cheese will run away! In addition, there is a delicious salad of roasted sweet potato, sweet pears and spicy red onion alongside. Maybe this will be your new favorite salad, because it's already ours!

Ingredients

For goat cheese salad
- 1 sweet potato
- 1 pear
- 1 Red onion
- 200 g goat cheese
- 60gwalnuts
- 2 Tea spoons honey
- 1 teaspoonthyme
- 50garugula
- 1 tbsp olive oil
- salt and pepper
- FOR THE DRESSING
- 1 tbsp olive oil
- 1 tbsp balsamic
- 1 teaspoon
- coarse-grained mustard

Preparation

1. Cut the sweet potato into small cubes, as well as the pear. Cut the red onion into thin strips and mix together with sweet potato, pear, olive oil, salt and pepper. Cook in the Airfryer for 20 minutes at 180 ° C.
2. In the meantime, the goat's cheese can be prepared. Cut this into 12 equal slices. Chop the walnuts and mix with the honey and thyme. Spread the walnut mixture evenly on the goat cheese slices with a spoon.
3. Wash the rocket, drain well and place in a large bowl. Once the sweet potatoes and pears are done, mix with the rocket and make a dressing of oil, vinegar and mustard. Mix well.
4. Finally, bake the goat's cheese slices in the airfryer; The airfryer is best lined with some baking paper. Bake the goat cheese for 3 minutes at 180 ° C, it may take longer!

5. Serve the salad on a plate and put a few slices of baked goat's cheese on it.

75   Perfect donuts from the airfryer

Donuts, these are sweet temptations. Either with a sweet glaze or filled, you can now find them everywhere where there are pastries. In principle, they are a sweeter version of our popular Berliners or pancakes - depending on where you come from. Allegedly, the early Dutch repatriates brought them to New York (then New Amsterdam). Anyone who has ever been to Holland knows the Oliebollen, which are very similar to our Berliners / pancakes / donuts. In the Airfryer you can prepare them without a fat bath or a guiltyconscience!

Ingredients

- 260 ml warm milk
- 55gsugar
- 1 pack yeast
- 2 eggs
- 140g butter
- 440g Flour
- 1/2 tsp salt
- melted butter to coat

For the glaze

- 200 g chocolate jam
- 50gwalnuts
- 30g
- coconut chips
- 200 g powdered sugar
- warm water

Preparation

1. For the dough, dissolve yeast, sugar and salt in lukewarm milk and let rest for 10 minutes.
2. Melt butter and add to the milk with the eggs. Add the flour and let it rest for 1 hour.

3. Sprinkle the tray with flour and roll out the dough (but not too thin). and let rest covered for 20 minutes again.
4. Put the donuts in the airfryer and brush with melted butter. Bake at 160 ° C for 6-8 minutes.
5. For the chocolate icing, melt the chocolate jam. Mix the icing sugar with water and stir to a creamy consistency. Now simply dip the finished donuts into the jam and sprinkle with coconut chips or walnuts - ready.

76 Three-grain bread from the Airfryer baking pan

For this we are known: delicious, grainy bread! For this we do not have to run to the bakery, but we can bake it quite comfortably at home; in the Airfryer. With this recipe, you will get two loaves of bread, baked one after the other using the baking-fry setting. This bread can be enjoyed with both savory and sweet toppings, whatever you like. We just thought about butter and cress. Delicious!

Ingredients

For 2 Loaves
- 1 kgWheat flour (type 550)
- 250 g spelt flour
- 750ml lukewarm water
- 1/2 cube butter
- 3,5 TL fresh yeast
- salt
- 1 teaspoonsugar
- 200 g Sunflower seeds
- 200 g linseed
- 100 g sesame
- some flour for kneading

Preparation

1. In a large bowl, dissolve the yeast cube in lukewarm water and stir with a whisk. Add salt and sugar and stir.
2. First add the wheat flour and fold in. Once the flour is combined with the water, add the spelt flour and knead into a smooth dough. Finally, knead the linseeds, sunflower seeds and sesame seeds. Cover the dough with a kitchen towel and leave for about an hour in a warm place until it has doubled.
3. Cut the dough in half, shape it into two loaves with a little flour, cut into it and let it sit, remembering to cover it, for another 20 minutes. Then coat with water, sprinkle with seeds and bake at 200 ° C for 35-40 minutes in the baking mold of the Airfryer.

77   Fish in sesame crust from the airfryer

Friday is fish day! Judith has come up with something very special for her and found a successful combination of light fish enjoyment and pleasantly warming oven vegetables. We used haddock for this dish, but any white fish is perfect! The sesame is in the foreground of this dish - it is the star, if you will. It gives the fish a pleasant crust that does not overpower the fish's own taste. The vegetables are added in the form of oil, creating an inimitable aroma. Fish was traditionally served in many places only on Fridays, we do not understand. With dishes like this, there should be fish every day!

Ingredients

for 4 persons
- 50g Sesame seeds
- 1 protein
- 1 Tbsp
- soy sauce
- 1 tbsp sesame oil
- 600g Fish (white, filet)
- 300g parsnips

- 250 g carrots
- 3 Garlic cloves
- 1 tbsp sesame oil
- Salt & pepper (to taste)
- 200ml vegetable stock

Preparation

1. First, the crust is prepared for the fish. For this, combine the sesame seeds, the egg white, soy sauce, and 1 tbsp sesame oil and set aside.
2. For the oven vegetables, peel the parsnips and carrots and cut into medium sized strips. Mix the garlic, 1 tbsp sesame oil, salt and pepper.
3. Place the vegetables in the airfryer at 180 ° C for 10 minutes. Then place the fish fillets on the vegetables and pour the sesame seeds liberally over them. Cook all together again for 13 minutes at 180 ° C.
4. Mince the vegetables with 200ml vegetable stock in a Food Processor to a puree. Serve the fish on the puree and enjoy!

78 Berry Crumble from the Airfryer

Berry Crumble is a simple sweet snack that can best be thought of as a kind of cake - just without dough. Sounds weird? it is not! It is perfect for a scoop of vanilla ice cream, yoghurt or simply to be consumed alone. The production is very simple and does not take much time. The scent of carmellising Crumble in the Airfryer is beguiling and the sweetness of the berries is the perfect flavor addition!

Ingredients For 4 Persons

- 110g oatmeal
- 50g grated coconut
- tbsp
- maple syrup
- 4 tbsp Sunflower oil
- 1/2 tsp cinnamon
- prize salt
- 30g almond flour
- 1 pck. TK berry mixture
- 3 tbsp maple syrup
- 1 tbsp lemon juice

- 1/2 tsp cinnamon

Preparation

1. For the crumble, mix oatmeal, coconut, maple syrup, sunflower oil, cinnamon, a pinch of salt, and almond flour and set aside.
2. Stir the remaining 3 tablespoons of maple syrup, lemon juice, cinnamon and the berry mixture and place in the baking mold of the Airfryer. Now add the crumble mass and place everything at 180 ° C for 15 minutes in the AirFryer. Finished!

79   Fluffy pancakes from the Airfryer baking dish

Don't we all love delicious, fluffy dough that tastes like a ski holiday? That's why we want to introduce you to this wonderful potato pancake recipe. In Austria, pots means as much as quark. This dessert tastes similar to cheesecake and is similar in style to Kaiserschmarrn, but differs slightly in the list of ingredients. Served with fresh raspberries and a little powdered sugar nothing can go wrong. The result: a fluffy, delicious potion dream!

Ingredients For 4 Servings

- 250 g Speisequark
- eggs
- 70g sugar
- 50gbutter
- 3 tbsp rum
- 3 tbsp semolina
- 1 pkvanilla sugar
- 50gfresh raspberries
- powdered sugar

Preparation

1. Stir egg yolks, butter and sugar until foamy and mix with quark, rum, semolina, and vanilla sugar.
2. Beat the egg whites until stiff and fold them under the dough.
3. Grease the baking mold of the Airfryer and fill with the dough. Bake at 180 C for 20 minutes, then pluck with two forks into small pieces and serve with fresh raspberries and some powdered sugar.

80 Beef roulades from the airfryer

Roulades have delighted people for a long time. Their first written record dates back to 1740, when they appeared as a recipe in a cookbook published in Amsterdam. To this day, they are not only popular in German-speaking countries, and with good reason. Because the filling is variable according to taste - the meat can be, for example, simply replaced by cabbage, so this dish can be prepared for vegetarians. But we left it classic and were very happy with the result! If the baking pan is used for the preparation, you can make a great sauce from the broth.

Ingredients For 4 Servings
- 800g Rinderrouladen
- Sour cucumbers
- slices of ham
- 4 tsp mustard
- Salt and pepper
- wooden sticks
- 4 small carrots
- 4 small potatoes
- 2 parsnips
- 1 Red onion
- 1 tbsp oil
- 1 teaspoonfresh rosemary

Preparation

1. Cut carrots, parsnips, potatoes and onions. Add oil, salt, pepper and rosemary, mix and cook at 180 °C for 10 minutes in the Philips Airfryer.
2. Now spread the beef roulades. Season with salt and pepper and brush with a teaspoon of mustard. Put a slice of ham on the roulade and cucumber on top. Roll up and fix with a wooden skewer. Kitchen yarn also works great for fixing.
3. Place the roulades on the pre-cooked vegetables and place in the hot air fryer at 180 °C for 15 minutes. Finished!

81 Eggplant chips from the Philips Airfryer

Eggplant fries are something very special! Quick to prepare, healthy, and with a unique texture. The possibilities are enormous with these vegetables, so you can, for example, rub them with salt to get the moisture out. After that, a dip in a tasty marinade - depending on your taste. We kept it rather simpler and fried it with a little sesame oil and sesame seeds.

Ingredients

- 500g aubergine
- 1 tbsp sesame oil
- 1 tbsp Sesame seeds
- Salt & pepper (to taste)

Preparation

1. Wash the aubergine and cut into strips.
2. Mix the aubergine strips with sesame oil, sesame seeds, salt and pepper and fry in the Airfryer at 180 ° C for 15 - 20 minutes - done!

82 Potato wedges from the Philips Airfryer

Potato wedges are especially something for those who want to get a little more out of their fries. More potato mass and often seasoned differently and served with sour cream they give the whole thing a completely different appearance than normal fries. We prepared them classically with some cooking oil and seasoned with salt & pepper.

Ingredients

- 500g Potatoes (boiling)
- 1 tbsp cooking oil
- Salt & pepper (to taste)

Preparation

1. Wash the potatoes and cut into slices. Potato wedges are usually prepared with peel, so you can save the peeling.
2. Now rinse the potato wedges in cold water to get the potato starch. This step is important so that they are also crispy.
3. Deep-frying is done twice. The first time at 120 ° C for 10 minutes in the airfryer. In the next step, the oil, salt and pepper are added and the columns are crisply fried at 180 ° C for 15 minutes. Finished!

83 Cordon Bleu from the Philips Airfryer

Everyone knows it and most love it: Cordon Bleu. Originally, Cordon Bleu was a blue ribbon on which hung the golden cross of the highest French knight's order. Over time, it has been used as a metaphor for elitism and has quickly become associated with high culinary art. The sophistication of Cordon Bleu then helped the court to his name. In your Airfryer you are guaranteed to succeed so well that your result deserves the name Cordon Bleu!

Ingredients

- chops
- 1 pck. Gouda cheese
- 1 pck. cooked ham
- eggs
- Flour (for breading)
- Panko breadcrumbs
- Salt pepper
- liquid butter

Preparation

1. Cut the chops in the middle so that you can unfold them. Note that the chop is still stuck on one side.
2. Beat the unfolded piece of meat under a plastic wrap with a meat tenderizer. Next, place a slice of gouda and boiled ham in the middle, season and chop.
3. Build up flour, eggs and breadcrumbs in a breading line and roll the folded pieces of meat one after the other in the individual bowls.
4. Brush the breaded Cordon Bleu with liquid butter and place in the Airfryer for 10 minutes at 200 ° C. As a side dish we have made a potato salad.

84 Camembert in the loaf of bread from the Philips Airfryer

Camembert in a loaf is the best of two worlds. One could well say it is a symbol of German-French friendship. German bread culture meets French cheese art. In any case, an excellent dish for friends and family! The fennel seeds and rosemary give the bread a delicious, hearty note that perfectly complements the cheese. It is done quickly and Camembert is available in every supermarket.

Ingredients

for 3-4 people

- 600g Wheat flour (type 405)
- 1 pck
- dry yeast
- 2 Teaspoons fennel seeds
- 1 tbsp honey
- 1 tbsp vinegar

- 450ml lukewarm water
- 1 pinch of sugar
- 2 Tea spoons salt
- 1 tbsp rosemary
- Camembert

Preparation

1. Mix yeast, salt, honey, and lukewarm water. Add vinegar, fennel and rosemary and mix. Finally, stir in the flour and mix well. Let the dough rest for one hour.
2. Put the dough in the pan and place the Camembert in the middle and press in a bit. Cover the cheese completely with the rest of the dough so that it is no longer visible. We sprinkled some rosemary on the crust as a decoration.
3. Put the bread in the airfryer at 200 ° C for 35 minutes. Serve immediately when it is ready, so that the cheese is still liquid.

85 Sweet potato fritters from the Philips Airfryer

Sweet potatoes have celebrated an unparalleled triumphal procession across the country. In the meantime, they are also found in the most unassuming restaurants; even in fast-food chains. Demand is just too big to ignore. Of course, we cannot withhold a corresponding recipe. You may have already prepared some - so you'll get another way with our recipe. Of course we could not resist a little trick.

Ingredients

- 500g sweet potatoes
- 1 tbsp olive oil
- cinnamon
- Salt & pepper (to taste)

Preparation

1. Wash the sweet potatoes, peel and cut into strips.
2. Pre-cook the sweet potato strips at 120 ° C for 10 minutes.
3. Now you can add the oil, cinnamon and, if needed, salt and pepper to the strips. Mix well with each other and place in the Airfryer at 180 ° C for 15 minutes.

86 Zucchini fries with peanut breading

Pommes is not the same potato that we want to prove once with this simple recipe! The possibilities here are virtually unlimited. We just kept it simple, but it's also a good idea to marinate the zucchini strips and let them go for a while. Ours were fried with peanut oil and got a light batter of minced roasted peanuts. Have fun experimenting!

INGREDIENTS

- 500g zucchini
- 1 tbsp peanut oil
- 1 Handful of roasted peanuts, minced
- Salt & pepper (to taste)

Preparation

1. Wash the zucchini and cut into strips.
2. Add peanut oil to the zucchini strips and also add the chopped peanuts. Put in the airfryer at 180 ° C for 15-20 minutes - done.

87 Vitelotte fries from the Philips Airfryer

Purple fries? Purple fries! Not only something unusual for the eye, but also perfect for the preparation of crispy fries, because the Vitelotte is a firm potato. It originates from the same homeland as the European potato, namely Peru and Bolivia. The taste is similar to sweet chestnuts but less sweet than our usual potato varieties. When you want to serve your family or guests a surprise, these potatoes are ideal. Especially for fries!

Ingredients

- 500g Vitelotte potatoes
- 1 tbsp rapeseed oil
- Salt & pepper (to taste)

Preparation

1. Wash the potatoes and cut into strips. You can also peel them if you feel like it.
2. Now rinse the vitelotto strips in cold water to get the potato starch. This step is important, so that the fries are nice and crispy.
3. Deep-frying is done twice. The first time, the fries go in the airfryer at 120 ° C for 10 minutes. This step is to cook them well inside. In the next step, the oil, salt and pepper are added and the fries are crisped at 180 ° C for 15 minutes. Finished!

88 Halloween snack from the Philips Airfryer

Soon the night of nights will come again. The night, which is different than the rest of the year. Strange figures bustle in the streets, shapes that you would not otherwise encounter. Halloween is coming soon! We have created a simple snack to celebrate this special night, which will put the little ones in the mood. Most of what you need for it, you have already at home. The preparation is done within a few minutes and it tastes good! The quantities in the recipe are somewhat vague, as it depends on how much you require.

Ingredients

- 1 pck. shortcrust
- 1 Block Cheddar
- 1 Glass of hot sausages
- 1 pck. almonds
- tomato paste
- 1 egg yolk

Preparation

1. Cut the cheddar into thin strips with a sharp knife. You must fit into a long-open hot sausage.
2. Cut the hot sausages lengthwise and place the cheddar inside.
3. Now cut the sausages with the cheddar into three pieces and roll them into the shortcrust pastry. Where the sausage was cut in, slightly compress the dough. This is how the "joints" of the fingers are created. Put some tomato paste on the top and an almond on top.
4. Brush the fingers with the egg yolk and place in the airfryer at 180 ° C for 12 minutes. Ketchup is recommended as a dip - it fits perfectly with the topic.

89 Warm pumpkin salad with cashew nuts and goat cheese

Salad is usually more associated with the warmer seasons. Especially in spring or summer, salads are booming because they are light and always fresh. Even though it gets cooler and a little bit more uncomfortable in the fall, it is still great for delicious salads. That's what we thought and so we prepared with our Airfryer a season-matching warm pumpkin salad.

Ingredients

- Pumpkin (diced)
- 1 tbsp oil
- prize

- cinnamon
- Salt and pepper
- 1 Red onion
- 1 teaspoonolive oil
- 1 tbsp maple syrup
- 1 teaspoondried thyme
- 1 Handful of cashew nuts
- 1 Handful of cranberries
- 1 Handful of basil
- 100 g soft goat cheese

Preparation

1. Marinate the diced pumpkin with the oil, a little salt and pepper and a pinch of cinnamon. Cook at 180 ° C for 20 minutes in the Airfryer.
2. In a pan, caramelise the red onion with a little olive oil and maple syrup. Once the onions are caramelized add cashew nuts, thyme, cranberries, basil, and goat's cheese. Season with salt & pepper.
3. In a bowl, mix the pans contents with the pumpkin from the airfryer and enjoy.

90   Original apple strudel from the Philips Airfryer

The Apple strudel! We do not know anyone who doesn't like it. The apple strudel is simply a legend! Originally from the Arabian area and later making its way to Europe, it was served as a marching food, food rather than a pastry. The reason for that was its long durability. These times are fortunately over. We have prepared ours to celebrate the Austrian national holiday, after all, the Austrians love their strudel so much that it is even good as a phrase. If something stretches so long that there is no end in sight, the Austrian says: "This is like a strudel" Thanks to the Philips Airfryer, however, the preparation is fast.

Ingredients for 2 servings
for the dough
- 440g Flour
- 60ml
- Sunflower oil
- 160ml water
- 1 egg
- salt

FOR THE FILLING
- 900g apples
- 120g
- granulated sugar
- 200 g bread crumbs
- 50gbutter
- 100 g raisins
- shotrum
- 1 teaspooncinnamon
- 40gButter (for brushing)

Preparation

1. Mix flour, egg, oil, salt and water together and knead into a dough.
2. Now heat the butter and sauté breadcrumbs in it.
3. Next, the apples can be peeled and cut into slices. Now mix the raisins, sugar, rum, cinnamon and the breadcrumbs.
4. Now roll out the dough on a floured kitchen towel and stretch into a rectangle and spread with melted butter.
5. Distribute the apple mixture in the upper third of the dough. The kitchen towel is ideal for curling up the strudel.
6. Brush the strudel again with liquid butter and bake at 160 ° C for 30 - 35 minutes. Serve with vanilla ice cream and enjoy.

91   Sweet potato slices with salsa from the airfryer

Kumpir (stuffed baked potatoes) are a typical Turkish fast food dish and are very popular in the big cities of this country. We took it and modified it a bit. Instead of a floury potato, we opted for sweet potato wedges and for the filling - or rather topping - a fiery salsa. Both work together very well and can be quickly and easily prepared without much effort!

   Ingredients For 2 Servings
for the potatoes
- 1 big sweet potato
- 1 tbsp
- olive oil
- 1/2 tsp Harissa

- 1/2 tsp salt
- 1/2 tsp pepper

FOR THE SALSA
- chili
- cherry tomatoes
- 1 Handful of basil
- 1 tbsp oil
- 1/2 tsp salt
- 1/2 tsp pepper
- spring onions

Preparation

1. The sweet potato should be cut into quarters and put in a bowl. Add olive oil, salt, pepper, and harissa and mix well with each other so that the sweet potatoes are evenly marinated. Cook the slices at 180 ° C in the Airfryer for 25 minutes.

2. Halve the tomatoes for the salsa and put them in a Food Processor along with some oil, chili, basil, salt, pepper and spring onions. Mix everything together for a short time. Take care that you do not chop too long, otherwise you'll get a pulp and not the typical lumpy salsa consistency.

3. Remove the sweet potato slices from the airfryer and serve with salsa. Finished!

Orange chicken fillets from the Philips Airfryer

As usual, we prepared our chicken breast fillets in the Philips Airfryer. Not just with salt, pepper and a few herbs, but with orange. The combination of sweet and savory gives the chicken a whole lot of charm. Try it yourself!

Ingredients

for 2 servings

- 2 Chicken breast fillets
- 2 tbsp honey
- 2 tbsp dried / fresh rosemary
- 1 tbsp olive oil

- Orange (juice & abrasion)
- Salt and pepper
- 1 onion

Preparation

1. The preparation of the chicken is very simple. Mix the fillets with the honey, rosemary, olive oil, salt and pepper. Add the rubbing and juice to half an orange and leave everything in the fridge for about 30 minutes.
2. Put the chicken in the airfryer at 180 ° C for 18 minutes with sliced onion and you're done! For example roasted sweet potatoes (from the Airfryer) are excellent as a side dish. But also rice and some salad is a good choice.

93   Bun Thit Nuong

This dish has everything we love about Vietnamese food. A wealth of flavors that harmonize beautifully with each other and a bowl full of great ingredients! The best thing about this dish: it's done in minutes! The only thing that takes time is the meat, which should be marinated for at least 30 minutes - better still overnight. The rest of the ingredients are cold rice noodles, fresh herbs such as coriander and / or mint, chopped roasted peanuts, sesame, spring onions and (pickled) carrot, cabbage and cucumber strips. What sounds like a lot of effort, is deceptive, because except for the meat, all ingredients are raw and only need to be cut. The rice noodles only need a few minutes in hot water.

Ingredients

FOR THE MEAT
- 400g Pork / beef
- 1 onion
- 2 tbsp sugar
- 2 tbsp Soy sauce
- 2 tbsp oil
- 1 tbsp Fish sauce
- 1-2 Garlic cloves
- 1 tbsp Lemongrass paste
- 1/2 tsp pepper
- Sesame and cilantro for garnish

TO SERVE
- 1 Portion of rice noodles

- 1 Handful of coriander
- 1 Handful of mint
- sliced cucumber and carrot strips
- 1 chopped spring onion
- chopped roasted peas

FOR THE DRESSING

- 6 tbsp water
- 2 tbsp sugar
- 2 tbsp
- lime juice
- 2 tbsp Fish sauce
- finely chopped garlic
- chopped chilli

Preparation

1. The marinade starts. Chop the onion and mix with the sugar, soy sauce, lemongrass paste, fish sauce, oil, garlic and some pepper. Cut the meat into thin strips and add to the marinade. If you have to go fast, it is enough to let the meat marinate for half an hour. Put the meat in the airfryer at 200 ° C for 13-15 minutes.
2. While the meat is cooking in the airfryer, the vegetables can be cut. Carrot should be cut in thin strips, cut the cucumber into slices, let the herbs go in whole. Roughly chop peanuts. The rice noodles need only a few minutes in hot, non-boiling water.
3. The dressing for the salad is super easy and done within 2 minutes. Mix together water, sugar, lime juice, fish sauce, garlic, and chilli - ready.
4. Put a portion of rice noodles in a bowl. Then we put in the meat. Next comes the vegetables and herbs. Now garnish with chopped peanuts, sesame seeds, and spring onions. The dressing can be added as desired.

Party shrimp skewers from the airfryer

Shrimp skewers are known from the Asian holiday or from the favorite Asian buffet. They are an excellent snack in between meals and can be made very easily. Thanks to the Philips Airfryer you can now enjoy them without a guilty conscience, because the AirFryer requires little oil to fry the breading crispy and gold-brown! As a dip, we have opted for a sweet and spicy version. This is very easy to prepare and lasts up to 2 weeks in the fridge. We thought the combination of crispy skewers and a sweetish dip with some fire was very successful and we would have liked to have had a little more of both! With the shrimp, it makes sense to take the largest possible - unfortunately we have only medium size.

Ingredients

FOR THE DIP

- 100 g sugar
- 2 tbsp water
- 125ml
- rice vinegar
- 1 tbsp Fish sauce
- 1 tbsp chilli flakes
- 1 clove of garlic
- 1/2 tsp Habanero Curry Powder (careful, very spicy)
- 1 lime
- 1 tbsp spring onions
- coriander

FOR THE SHRIMP

- 500g Shrimp (the bigger the better)
- 2-3eggs
- Sesame, salt & pepper
- Flour
- Panko breadcrumbs
- 1 pck. wooden skewers

Preparation

1. We start with the dip as it is cooked in a pan and then we should allow it to cool down. Mix the sugar and water in a bowl to a sandy consistency and place in a pan. Cook on high heat until the mass assumes a light golden color. Now add

vinegar, fish sauce, chilli flakes, garlic, and curry powder immediately and cook while stirring until it has a syrupy consistency. Set aside and let cool.

2. Peel the prawns, press down on a work surface with their legs down and skewer them lengthwise. Once all are skewered, the breading line can be prepared.
3. In a bowl of flour and then in a second give the eggs and whisk. Fill the third bowl with panko breadcrumbs, sesame seeds, salt & pepper and mix well. Roll the shrimp skewers first in the flour, then in the eggs and finally in the panko. Fry at 200 ° C for 8 minutes until golden brown.
4. Once the prawns are done, pour the dip into a bowl, add the juice of half a lime and garnish with some cilantro and spring onions. You can also use the juice of a whole lime, but the consistency of the dips then becomes more fluid.

95 Filled burger from the airfryer

This is not for the faint of heart, a true heavyweight among the Burgers! For some, it may be a bit too much of a good thing and for others will bring real excitement to their eyes. This burger - aka the Colossus of Airfryers - is filled with everything you like. Sheathed in crispy bacon and topped with real buffalo mozzarella. We have filled our colossus with a mixture of red onions, red pointed peppers, and brown mushrooms - you are here as the doors open!

Ingredients

for 2 burgers
- 500g Beef minced beef
- big mushrooms
- 2 small red pointed paprika
- 1 Red onion
- 1 Handful of basil
- 1 Handful of dried tomatoes
- 1 teaspoonPaprika powder rose sharp

- Slices of bacon
- Salt pepper
- oil
- 2 Burger buns
- 1 Ball buffalo mozzarella

Preparation

1. Chop onions, peppers and mushrooms and sauté in a pan with a little oil until everything has lost some of its volume. Season with salt and pepper and set aside.
2. For the burgers mix the minced meat with chopped basil, dried tomatoes, salt, pepper and paprika powder. Form a large ball out of it and divide into 2 equal parts.
3. Press the two balls with a beer bottle or can in the middle, creating a kind of chamber. Fill both chambers with the mushroom, onion and pepper mixture and cover with the mozzarella. Wrap it all up with the bacon and put the two burgers in the airfryer for 12 minutes at 180 ° C.

96   Our absolute favorite waffle recipe!

Waffles are a pastry made of flour and water in their simplest form. They are a timeless classic. Not only because they have been tasting great for centuries - their first mention dated back a good 1000 years - but also because they delight us from childhood to old age. A waffle makes you love, a waffle makes you happy. We appreciate that as much as others do. They appear in many regions, in the most varied forms and with the most diverse recipes. Whether with hot cherries, vanilla ice cream, icing sugar, or simply served: the waffle is a true perennial favorite!

INGREDIENTS

for four waffles
- eggs
- 125g sugar
- 1 pck. vanilla sugar
- 125g butter
- 2 Teaspoons baking powder
- 250 g Flour
- 250ml milk
- 1 TBSP oil

- 1 pinch of salt

Preparation

1. Mix eggs, sugar and vanilla into a mixture. Then add the diced butter and fold in briefly.
2. Now add the baking powder, flour, milk and a pinch of salt and mix. In your Airfryer, the waffles are baked golden brown within 12 minutes at 160 ° C. Let the waffles cool a little before you release them from the mold.

97 Galette from the airfryer

"Galette, what's that?" was the first reaction from some in the team. The answer to this question could not be easier, because a galette is nothing else than the hearty version of the famous and popular crepe. Native to Brittany, the dough is traditionally made only from buckwheat flour, salt and water. As usual, we have deviated from the original and have put our own stamp on it. The dough is now a bit crisp and is similar to a quiche. For the filling we stayed with something autumnal and decided on a mix of pears, walnuts, and soft goat's cheese. The result, we agree, would bring praise even to the proudest Breton!

Ingredients

for 2 galettes

for the dough
- 110g wheat flour
- 110g
- spelled flour
- 125ml cold water
- 150g cold butter

- 1 teaspoon salt
- 1/2 tsp vinegar

FOR THE FILLING

- 2 pears
- 2 Red onions
- 1 tbsp fresh rosemary
- 50g walnuts
- 1 tbsp oil
- 100 g soft goat cheese
- Salt pepper

Preparation

1. Mix the ingredients for the dough in a bowl, then knead well by hand and chill for 1 hour.
2. The filling can be prepared shortly before the end of the cooling time. To do this, heat the oil in a pan. Fry the onions and pears together with the rosemary and walnuts. Season with salt and pepper. Then set aside.
3. Now the Galettes can be prepared. Roll out the dough on a floured work surface into 2 equal parts. Place the filling from the pan evenly in the middle of the two dough pies and spread some goat's cheese on top. Now just fold the edges of the flatbread over the filling so that the middle stays open.
4. The Galettes cook at 180 ° C for 20 minutes in the Airfryer. After 15 minutes baking time, the dough can be coated with a little water.

98 Mediterranean aubergine with Tahini dressing

Who needs meat when there are these wonderful eggplants? They not only taste different Mediterranean spices, but thanks to the pistachio nuts are deliciously crunchy and thanks to the Tahini dressing wonderfully creamy. This dish can be made very fast, is easy to prepare and does not require a long list of ingredients. Throw on an apron and go!

Ingredients

- 2 small eggplants
- 2 Tea spoons salt
- 3 tbsp olive oil
- 1 teaspoonpaprika
- 1 TEASPOON dried rosemary

- 1 teaspoon Falafel spice (caraway, coriander, ginger)
- 1 clove of garlic
- 50g roasted pistachios, roughly chopped
- 1 tbsp fresh rosemary, finely chopped
- 60ml Tahini
- Lemon, pressed
- 3 tbsp water
- 1 pinch of salt
- 1/2 tsp Ground caraway
- 1/4 tsp Coriander, ground
- 1 clove of garlic
- 1 teaspoon Sesame, for garnish

Preparation

1. Cut the aubergines lengthwise into steaks and place for 30 minutes in 2 teaspoons of salt.
2. In a small bowl, combine olive oil with the chopped garlic clove, dried rosemary, falafel spice and paprika.
3. After 30 minutes, dab the aubergines with a paper or kitchen towel to reduce excess salt and liquid.
4. Marinate the aubergines in the oil mixture and then cook in the Airfryer at 200 degrees for 13-15 minutes.
5. Mix the Tahini in the KitchenAid Mini Food Processor with cumin, coriander, a pinch of salt, the juice of half a lemon and a clove of garlic. Meanwhile, add some water through the small hole in the lid of the Food Processor to get a creamy, smooth dressing consistency.
6. Arrange the aubergine slices on a plate and garnish with a little Tahini dressing and the chopped pistachios and fresh rosemary.

99 Crispy sushi

Who does not love, probably the most internationally famous Japanese dish. Whether filled with different types of vegetables, fish, tofu or even meat, one thing is clear: there is versatility in sushi. For the preparation, special sushi rice is used, which must be thoroughly washed so that it does not stick more than necessary. Then the nori leaves are covered with the rice to about three quarters, to then add the desired coating such as fresh salmon, avocado, mango, cucumber or carrot.

When filling the sushi rolls the imagination knows no bounds! This recipe includes classic stuffed sushi, but the rice flour sesame breading makes them special. Try it!

INGREDIENTS

- 300g Sushi Rice
- 1 tbsp sugar
- 60ml
- Rice wine vinegar
- 1 cucumber
- 2 carrots
- 1 ripe avocado
- Nori sheets
- big tiger shrimps
- 175g rice flour
- 3 eggs
- pinch turmeric
- 3 tbsp sesame
- 100 g breadcrumbs
- Oil for spraying
- Wasabi
- soy sauce

Preparation

1. Thoroughly wash the rice in a colander and then boil in 450ml cold water and 1 teaspoon of salt. Once the rice cooks, the temperature can be reduced. Pour the cooked rice into a bowl and let it cool in the open.
2. Once the rice is lukewarm, add the rice wine vinegar and sugar and a pinch of salt and stir well. Chill the rice for at least 30 minutes.
3. Halve the avocado, remove the core, spoon out the inside and cut into strips. Quarter the cucumber and carrots and cut into strips as well. Make sure that the strips are no longer than the width of the Nori leaves.
4. Wash the tiger prawns, peel them, cut them lengthwise into strips and sprinkle with some lime juice to pre-heat them.
5. Spread the bamboo mat (alternatively it is also possible with aluminum foil), put a nori leaf on it and distribute 1 cm thick rice on it. There must be some

space above, leaving about 1/4 of the area clear. Press the rice a bit flat and cover each with carrot, cucumber, avocado and tiger prawns. Using the bamboo mat, roll the nori leaf and press the end of the leaf firmly to the sushi roll with a little water.

6. Fill the rice flour into the first bowl, up to the breading line. In the second bowl the eggs can be whisked. Finally, mix the breadcrumbs with sesame and turmeric and prepare as the last stop on the breading line. First cut the sushi rolls in half and then toss in the rice flour, then add to the egg mixture and then cover with the sesame breadcrumb mixture.

7. Lay out the basket of the airfryer with baking paper and place the sushi rolls on it. Sprinkle with a little oil and bake at 200 degrees for 10-12 minutes until golden-brown. Cut the ready-baked rolls into pieces and serve with some wasabi and soy sauce.

100 Stuffed tomatoes from the Philips Airfryer

Filled tomatoes? Who is doing that? We are, because this dish is an absolute asset to everyone - guaranteed! Easier to prepare than it sounds, delicious and incredibly healthy. This is due above all to the lentils, which are rich in iron, magnesium and vitamins. Except for the lentils, which must already be cooked, the complete dish can be prepared in the Philips Airfryer. This not only saves time but also a lot of washing up! It can be served as a snack or as a full meal, for example with a crispy salad as a side dish. But even a few slices of garlic bread are excellent.

INGREDIENTS

for 2 people
- medium sized tomatoes
- 2 Garlic cloves
- onion
- 150g lenses
- 90ml Tomato sauce
- 1 tbsp olive oil
- 1 teaspoonbalsamic
- 2 tbsp herbs of Provence

- 30g grated almonds
- Basil to decorate

Preparation

1. Fry the onion, garlic and Provence herbs in olive oil in the Airfryer for 5 minutes at 200 ° C. We used the baking pan for this.
2. In the meantime, cut a slice under the tomato's stalk and then hollow out with a teaspoon. Put the pulp in a separate bowl and chop large pieces.
3. Now the pulp can be added to the fried onions. The lentils and almonds are now also added. Stir everything and fry for 5 minutes at 200 ° C.
4. Now fill the tomatoes with the mix from the airfryer. It will not all fit in the tomatoes, but that's no problem. Just mix the rest with some tomato sauce and balsamic, put the tomatoes on top and cook everything at 200 ° C for 10 minutes. Finally, decorate with basil and Parmesan.

101 Sweet bacon muffins with maple syrup

That sweet and salty fit together well, we now know this - chocolate and ice, sea salt and caramel, so "Salted Caramel", has finally arrived with us. The muffins are as always nicely juicy in the airfryer and also the bacon we have cooked to a crisp directly from frozen in the AirFryer.

Ingredients

Ingredients for 18 muffins

- 50g Butter
- 100g sugar
- 2 Owner
- ¼ Backsoda / Natron
- Pck natural vanilla flavor
- 240ml milk
- Shot of maple syrup
- 60ml vegetable oil
- 70g Brown sugar
- 1 1/2 TL baking powder
- 3/4 TL salt
- 280g Flour
- 125g bacon

Preparation

1. Remove the airfryer basket and replace the grille with the grill plate. Replace the basket, spread the bacon on the griddle and fry at 200 ° C for 7 minutes until the cubes are crispy-brown.
2. In a large bowl, stir butter, oil and sugar together until the sugar has completely dissolved. Set the hand mixer to medium and stir in the eggs one at a time.
3. Then add baking soda, salt and vanilla flavor.
4. Prepare the flour and milk and stir in two tablespoons, until a smooth dough is formed.
5. Provide 9 silicone muffin cups and fill each one to about 1 cm below the rim. Sprinkle each muffin evenly with bacon and drizzle with about 1 tablespoon of maple syrup.
6. Place molds in the airfryer and fry at 160 ° C for 14 minutes.
7. Allow the muffins to cool slightly and pour over some maple syrup before serving.

102 Apple rings - a round thing

Autumn is coming. The summer was long, warm and very beautiful - nevertheless, we are starting to get excited about the most colorful of the seasons. One reason for this is the freshly picked apples that are now in season. So to make the transition a little more pleasant, we decided on a light and very simple snack: apple rings with a crunchy nut crust. Prepared, of course, in our beloved Philips Airfryer XXL. We used the grill of the party kit, because we were able to bake twice the amount of apple rings and still had enough space without them sticking together. For breading we used the breading set, which is also available in our shop. Our kitchen thanked us! The recipe is of course individually customizable, depending on taste. We were impressed with the results, because the rings are great both warm with custard and cold! A great snack, which you can just leave on the kitchen table!

INGREDIENTS

Ingredients for 2 servings
- 2 apples
- 3-4 EL Flour
- 1/2 TL baking powder
- 1 TL cinnamon
- 1 EL honey
- 4 EL sugar

- 150g Nussmix

Preparation

1. Thoroughly wash the apples, core them and cut into slices of approx. 0.5cm thick. They should not be cut too short, but too thick is not a problem. Optionally, the apple slices could also be drizzled with a little lemon juice.
2. For the dough, mix an egg with flour and baking powder. We added some honey to sweeten it. It is important that a tough mass is formed, which adheres well to the apple and does not drip. If the dough is too firm, it can simply be loosened up with a dash of milk. Put the mass in a bowl up to the breading line.
3. Coarsely chop nuts for the breading. We chose a mix of hazelnuts and almonds. Optionally, the nuts can also be roasted briefly in the Airfryer, so they have a stronger flavor. Put the mix in a pan up to the breading line.
4. Now rub the apples with cinnamon and sugar and place in the dough, so that they are covered by a uniform film. Now simply add to the nut mix and bake at 180 ° C for 12 minutes. It is advisable to spray the basket and the grill with a little oil, so that nothing sticks.

103 Salmon with fennel and orange from the airfryer

Salmon is usually prepared as a hearty dish., with butter and many herbs. We changed our mind this time and baked the salmon with fennel, which is currently in season, and fruity orange in the Philips Airfryer XXL. The result was very promising, because the slightly aniseed taste of the vegetables in combination with the sweet-fruity flavor of the orange complements the fish perfectly. The dish is great as a light lunch or dinner, and can be served with rice or a salad. The great thing about salmon: the leftovers can also be eaten cold the next day and used up, for example, as a sandwich. Or eaten for breakfast with cream cheese.

INGREDIENTS

Ingredients for 2 servings

- Tablespoons olive oil
- 1 orange
- 300g salmon
- 1 fennel
- 1 Bunch dill
- Salt and pepper

Preparation

1. Cut the orange and fennel into even slices and season with a dash of olive oil and some salt and pepper. Bake at 160 ° C for 10 minutes.
2. Now put the dill, fennel, and the oranges together and embed the salmon on them. Season again with a little salt, pepper and olive oil and grate some orange peel on the fish. Bake again for 10 minutes at 160 ° C in the Airfryer and it is ready!

104 Tornado potatoes with bacon and cheese from the airfryer

We love potatoes because they are so incredibly versatile. This recipe is another impressive testament to this and will delight both children and adults alike. Many will know the Tornado Potatoes or Spiral Potatoes from the Fair where they are commonly found. With the Philips Airfryer you no longer need to wait for the next fair or street party, because you can prepare them at home! We refined it with some bacon and cheese and served them with an herbal quark dip. Particularly suitable for birthdays of the little ones or if you do not have much at home, because potatoes are always there.

INGREDIENTS

for 2 servings
- 2 potatoes
- 50g Speck
- 50g cheese
- Herbs, quark & parsley

Preparation

1. Pierce a potato with a wooden skewer in the middle. Replace the wooden spit with a metal one and cut it diagonally with a knife, so that the potato can be pulled apart as a spiral. Leave the metal skewer in to fry the potatoes.
2. Wash the starch from the potatoes under running water. Then lay out on the grill pan of the Airfryer and fry at 120 ° C for 15 minutes. Then inject with a little oil and cook for another 10 minutes at 180 ° C in the AirFryer.
3. Put some grated cheese and bacon cubes on the spirals, garnish with a little rosemary and fry for another 3 minutes at 180 ° C. Now the potatoes can be plastered with a dip of your choice.

105 Poached eggs from the airfryer

The breakfast egg, man's best friend at an early hour! It usually comes cooked as fried eggs cooked only on one sider, then called Sunny Side Up. But why settle for a standard egg when the Philips Airfryer offers you so many more options without much effort? Exactly, we thought so too! So learn how to make a poached egg from our favorite hot air fryer.

Ingredients

- for 1 slice of bread
- Avocado
- 1 clove of garlic
- 3-6 Cherrytomaten
- 1L boiling water
- 50ml vinegar
- 1-2 EL Sriracha Sauce
- Parsley, salt & pepper

Preparation

1. To poach the eggs, pour 1l boiling water into the baking mold of the airfryer and add the vinegar. Then carefully insert the eggs into the liquid and if necessary hold them together with a spoon. Cook for 3-5 minutes in the Airfryer at 200 ° C.
2. For the spread, chop an avocado, garlic and tomatoes. Mix with a little Sriracha sauce, olive oil and a little salt. Serve everything on a slice of toasted bread and garnish with parsley and lemon zest.

106 Burger dumplings from the Airfryer: crazy and damn delicious

We of Generation YES are absolute fans of dumplings. Whether hearty with meat, or with fish and vegetables, or with sweet jam, we are always over the moon when there are dumplings. Seriously, whoever came up with the idea of filling dough balls with goodies is nothing short of a genius! The same is true of sandwiches or burgers. We have a slightly fancier recipe for you this time and are convinced that it will put a big smile on your face. Because we combine the best of two very interesting and diverse worlds to introduce you to the slightly different snack: the Big Mac Mini Balls! The Philips Airfryer impressively demonstrates its all rounder qualities again and makes it easy for you because you need nothing more than the versatile AirFryer. The dumplings are ideal as a finger food for parties or to make sense of the last remnants of the homemade pizza dough.

Ingredients

for 6 balls
- 300g Hack
- 2 onions

- somethingSalt pepper
- 100g Pizzateig
- 100g Bacon
- 50gMayo
- 150g Cheddar
- 50gliquid butter
- 1 Handful of sesame seeds
- 1 Handful of sour cucumbers

Preparation

1. Put the minced meat and chopped onions in the grill pan of your Philips Airfryer. Season with salt and pepper, mix everything and bake for 5 minutes at 200 ° C.
2. From the pizza dough, punch out circular surfaces - e.g. with a glass - and top them with a little ground beef. Do not add too much meat here, as there is a piece of bacon, some mayo and a small slice of cheddar cheese still to go on top. Now pack everything, so that everything concludes well and you have a bulging dough ball.
3. Now put the Big Mac Mini Balls on some baking paper in the grill pan of your Airfryer and coat them with some liquid butter. Sprinkle the balls with some sesame seeds and bake for 7 minutes at 180 ° C. Now dice the sour cucumbers, skewer on toothpicks and put them into the finished dumplings.

107 Cheese volcano from the Airfryer - the sociable snack

Although I'm not really a big cheese fan, this dish convinced me completely otherwise. Especially for a relaxing evening with friends, family or neighbors this snack is perfect. The triplets are ideal for dipping in the cheese crater of our volcano and the crispy pizza dough coating around it gives the whole thing the necessary crunch. Garlic in the cheese and potatoes rounds off the dish. The trick here is that you can prepare the cheese volcano and triplets comfortably together in the Airfryer. So everything is cooked evenly and gently in the Philips AirFryer and you can meanwhile devote your full attention to your guests, without having to disappear for a long time in the kitchen. I love such dishes.

INGREDIENTS

for 8 persons
- 2 Camembert
- Garlic cloves

- 1 Pizzateig
- 300g triplets
- 2 EL olive oil
- Salt & fresh thyme

Preparation

1. First, the Camembert is prepared in batter. For this purpose, you separate both surfaces of a piece, but leave the second piece of cheese to a turn. Stack the two Camembert pieces on top of each other and put 3 toes of garlic in the cheese.
2. Roll out your pizza dough and place the Camembert, with the remaining surface up, in the middle of the dough. Here, bought doughs are just as good as homemade doughs. Next, wrap the cheese in the dough so that everything locks up well.
3. The cheese in the batter comes embedded on baking paper in the grill pan of the Airfryer. The triplets can now be placed around it. Drizzle some olive oil over the potatoes and add 2 cloves of garlic. Salt everything and bake at 160 ° C for 25 minutes. At the end of the baking time, cut away the pastry top and decorate the contents with a little thyme.

108 Samosas - Crunchy, Spicy, Tasty

I'm sure you've eaten samosas with an Indian meal as an appetizer: crunchy bags filled with roasted vegetables, peas and potatoes or minced meat, for example. For the "Samosa AirFryern Happening" we decided on a classic potato-pea-mince filling, the bags we have hot-fried as usual with little fat in the airfryer.

INGREDIENTS

for 16 pieces

- 300g Flour
- 5 EL vegetable oil
- 1 TL Salt (heaped)
- 145ml water
- 1 Bunch dill
- 1 big potato
- 2 EL vegetable oil
- 1 onion
- 1 Garlic cloves
- 1 TL cumin

- 1 TL Coriander (ground)
- 1/2 TL cinnamon
- 1 rote Chili
- sea-salt
- 150g peas
- 1 bay leaf
- 450g ground beef
- 1 EL ginger
- 1 TL Curcuma
- 1 TL Chili
- 1 TL cardamom
- fresh coriander & pepper

Preparation

1. Boil potatoes and peas and process them with a potato masher to a lumpy mass. Set the mass aside and let it cool.
2. In the meantime, stir together a bowl of flour, salt, oil, and water and then knead well with your hands for at least 10 minutes to form a smooth dough. Cover the dough and let rest for about 30 minutes.
3. Peel the onions and garlic and finely chop. Put the grill plate in the basket of the airfryer and fry the minced meat with onions and garlic at 180 ° C for 7 minutes.
4. Use bay leaves, turmeric, cumin, chilli powder, cardamom, pepper, salt and cinnamon to make a spice mixture in a mortar and pestle.
5. Cut the chili into thin rings and mix the potato mixture with the fried minced meat, grated ginger, chilli pepper and spice mixture.
6. On a lightly floured work surface, roll out a small piece of dough (8 in total) in a thin circular shape, halve the circle, turn over one third of the semicircle, brush with water and fold the second third into a school bag shape.
7. Fill the resulting bags with the potato mixture and fresh coriander leaves, leave about 1.5cm space above. Brush the doormat with water, press in and press firmly so that the bag is closed.
8. Insert the basket back into the airfryer, place 8 samosas into the airfryer, spray with oil and fry at 180 ° C for 15 minutes.

109 Tornado potatoes with bacon and onions

Tornado potatoes are the latest trend in airfryer skies, because there is virtually no work to prepare this dish, but crispy chips, melted cheese and crispy bacon can be enjoyed at once.

Of course, you can also enjoy the potatoes vegetarian or vegan and just fill them with cheese or herbs of your choice, and off to the AirFryer! The perfect snack for all occasions.

Ingredients

for 2 servings

- 2 big potatoes
- 50ggrated cheese
- rosemary
- 50gdiced bacon

Preparation

1. Wash the potatoes and skewer them lengthwise. Using a sharp kitchen knife, cut into a spiral on the wooden stick. If present, spit the potatoes on metal skewers, pull apart and rinse thoroughly under cold water until the water is clear.
2. Place the potatoes in the Airfryer and dry at 120 ° C for 15 minutes.
3. After 15 minutes, spray dried potatoes with oil and fry at 180 ° C for 10 minutes.
4. Then fill the potatoes with bacon and cheese and sprinkle with rosemary. We did not salt them additionally here, as we have a strong sour cream for dipping.
5. Cook the potatoes for a further 3 minutes at 180 ° C - the sour cream will be a perfect match!

110 Broccoli croquettes

Fortunately, Panko breadcrumbs have arrived in almost every supermarket, and if you have not tried them yet, it's high time. Instead of breadcrumbs, Panko consists of larger pieces of roasted white bread, it takes less fat when cooked in the Airfryer, but becomes extra crispy. They are perfect for delicious broccoli croquettes from the AirFryer! The croquettes are great as a standalone meal, but also makes a good side dish.

Ingredients

for 15 pieces

- 500g broccoli
- 3 tbsp bread crumbs
- 1 small onion

- Flour
- 1 teaspoonnutmeg
- 100 g grated cheese
- 1 clove of garlic
- eggs
- Panko breadcrumbs, salt & fresh pepper

Preparation

1. Boil the broccoli in lightly salted water, cut into small pieces and place in a bowl.
2. Peel garlic and onions, finely chop the garlic, dice the onions and add to broccoli with cheese, 2 eggs, breadcrumbs and spices. Mix all ingredients with a wooden spoon to a mass.
3. A Panierstraße build and each fill a tray with flour, egg and Panko. Salt, pepper and whisk the egg.
4. Provide a bowl with lukewarm water, cut off with one tablespoon of coconut from the mass, bring into shape and roll first in flour, then egg, then panko. In between, if necessary, moisten the hands in the bowl.
5. Place the croquettes in the airfryer, sprinkle lightly with oil and fry at 200 ° C for 10 minutes.

111 English breakfast

English breakfast is enjoyed often by me as a brunch - I confess, I also like to eat it for dinner. The thick streaky bacon becomes crunchy in the Airfryer, the sausages crisp and brown and mushrooms and tomatoes are perfectly grilled in the hot air fryer. If all these delicacies are on the plate, an English breakfast is simply irresistible!

Ingredients

Ingredients for 2 persons

- 1 big tomato

- Nuremberg roast sausages
- thick slices of bacon
- fresh pepper
- 4 mushrooms
- 2 eggs
- 1 Can of baked beans
- toast

Preparation

1. Wash and slice the tomato, clean mushrooms and quarter them. Insert the grill plate from the grill kit into the basket of the Airfryer.
2. Put the sausages, bacon, tomato slices, and mushrooms on the grill plate, and spray the mushrooms with oil. Grill everything at 180 ° C for 10 minutes.
3. Put the grid back into the basket, put the baking tin in the airfryer and put in the beans. Spread the beans flat with a spoon and put 2 eggs on top.
4. Fry again at 180 ° C for 10 minutes.
5. Serve everything on a plate with toast and butter.

112 Frikandeln Speciaal - Dutch meat rolls with mayo and onions

Hard-core fry lovers and fry friends, we do not have much to explain now, because Frikandeln are the hit for the AirFryer. "I'm going over to Holland, should I bring something?" is always first answered with "fricandles", and in the Netherlands you can get the meat rolls at practically every snack bar and in every supermarket. "Speciaal" means nothing more than some ketchup, a lot of mayo and a few fresh onion cubes, if you do not already know it: Be sure to try it!

Ingredients

Ingredients for 5 rolls
- 500g minced meat
- 1 tbsp chicken broth
- 50ml milk
- 1 tbsp Parpikapulver
- 1 teaspoon curry powder
- 1 eggs
- 1 tbsp Ketchup
- 150g Chicken breast

- 1 Slices of toasted bread
- 1 teaspoon nutmeg
- 1 teaspoon chilli flakes
- 1 teaspoon garlic powder
- fresh parsley
- pepper
- onion
- mayonnaise

Preparation

1. Dissolve 1 tablespoon of instant chicken stock in 100ml of boiling water and chill. Cut the chicken breast very small with a sharp kitchen knife. Pour the toast in a bowl with the milk and set aside.
2. In a good blender or multi-sizer, puree the chicken, egg and spices for a few seconds. Add toasted bread into the blender, add cooled broth and puree everything again until a fine meatloaf is produced. Please do not purée too long, so that the meat does not begin to cook in the crusher or the mixture becomes too liquid. Transfer the meat for about 10 minutes into the freezer.
3. On a work surface, lay out a piece of cling film about 30cm long. Make 2 generous tablespoons of meatloaf on the foil in roll form, wrap the sausage tightly and turn the ends as you would for a candy. Wrap 5 meat rolls and place in the refrigerator.
4. Put a pot of water on the stove and heat to about 85 ° C (the water should not boil yet). Put the meat rolls in the foil in the water and let them steep for 8 minutes. Remove the rolls, allow to cool briefly and unwind.
5. Place the rolls in the airfryer, spray with oil and fry at 200 ° C for 12 minutes until crispy brown.
6. Peel the onion and cut into small pieces. Cut the frikandel into half length on a plate, fill with ketchup and mayonnaise and serve with onions.

www.ingramcontent.com/pod-product-compliance
Lightning Source LLC
Chambersburg PA
CBHW081400070526
44583CB00020B/2607